Improving
Dementia
Long-Term Care

A Policy Blueprint

Regina A. Shih

Thomas W. Concannon

Jodi L. Liu

Esther M. Friedman

The research in this report was produced within RAND Health and RAND Labor and Population, units of the RAND Corporation. This report results from the RAND Corporation's Investment in People and Ideas program. Support for this program is provided, in part, by the generosity of RAND's donors and by the fees earned on client-funded research.

Library of Congress Cataloging-in-Publication Data

Shih, Regina A., author.
  Improving dementia long-term care : a policy blueprint / Regina A. Shih, Thomas W. Concannon, Jodi L. Liu, Esther M. Friedman.
      p. ; cm.
  Includes bibliographical references.
  ISBN 978-0-8330-8630-3 (pbk. : alk. paper)
I. Concannon, Thomas W., author. II. Liu, Jodi L., author. III. Friedman, Esther M., 1976- author. IV. Rand Corporation, issuing body. V. Title.
  [DNLM: 1. Aged—United States. 2. Dementia—therapy—United States. 3. Long-Term Care—United States. 4. Quality Improvement—United States. WT 155]
  RC521
  362.1968'3—dc23
                                                                                            2014023140

Support RAND—make a tax-deductible charitable contribution at www.rand.org/giving/contribute.html

RAND® is a registered trademark.

Cover design by Peter Soriano

© Copyright 2014 RAND Corporation

RAND OFFICES
SANTA MONICA, CA • WASHINGTON, DC
PITTSBURGH, PA • NEW ORLEANS, LA • JACKSON, MS • BOSTON, MA
CAMBRIDGE, UK • BRUSSELS, BE
www.rand.org

Preface

In 2013, Michael D. Hurd, the director of the RAND Center for the Study of Aging, and his colleagues published landmark research in the *New England Journal of Medicine* on the monetary costs of dementia in the United States.[1] They estimated that dementia, with costs of $159 billion to $215 billion annually, takes a higher economic toll on the nation than heart disease or cancer. Based on the significant implications of this information, Michael D. Rich, president and chief executive officer of the RAND Corporation, tasked a team of investigators to consider public policies that improve long-term services and supports for persons with dementia and the family and friends who provide care for them, often at the cost of the caregiver's own health status and financial assets. With the generous support of a gift from longtime RAND benefactor Charles J. Zwick and RAND Health, this study builds on the work of Hurd and others at RAND with nonpartisan, objective research to propose a blueprint for policy options identified by a range of stakeholders. RAND then evaluated these policy options on impact and feasibility metrics. This blueprint offers policy options to help decisionmakers improve the delivery of long-term services and supports, to bolster the workforce that provides those services and supports, and to outline financing solutions, with a focus on the needs of persons with dementia and their caregivers. These policy options serve as a foundation upon which to engage stakeholders in a larger debate and to build consensus on a set of policy recommendations.

This report results from the RAND Corporation's Investment in People and Ideas program. Support for this program is provided, in part, by the generosity of RAND's donors and by the fees earned on client-funded research. The research presented herein was conducted jointly by RAND Health and RAND Labor and Population, divisions of the RAND Corporation. Profiles of RAND Health and RAND Labor and Population, abstracts of their publications, and ordering information can be found at http://www.rand.org/health and http://www.rand.org/labor.html.

Abstract

In 2010, 15 percent of Americans older than age 70 had dementia, and the number of new dementia cases among those 65 and older is expected to double by the year 2050. As the baby boomer generation ages, many older adults will require dementia-related long-term services and supports (LTSS). This blueprint is the only national document to date that engages local, state, and national stakeholders to specifically focus on policy options at the intersection of dementia and LTSS.

The authors undertook five major tasks that resulted in a prioritized list of policy options and research directions to help decisionmakers improve the dementia LTSS delivery system, workforce, and financing. These were to

1. Identify weaknesses in the LTSS system that may be particularly severe for persons with dementia.
2. Review national and state strategies addressing dementia or LTSS policy.
3. Identify policy options from the perspective of a diverse group of stakeholders.
4. Evaluate the policy options.
5. Prioritize policy options by impact and feasibility.

Stakeholders identified 38 policy options. RAND researchers independently evaluated these options against prespecified criteria, settling on 25 priority options. These policy options can be summarized into five objectives for the dementia LTSS system:

1. Increase public awareness of dementia to reduce stigma and promote earlier detection.
2. Improve access to and use of LTSS.
3. Promote high-quality, person- and caregiver-centered care.
4. Provide better support for family caregivers of people with dementia.
5. Reduce the burden of dementia LTSS costs on individuals and families.

This policy blueprint provides a foundation upon which to build consensus among a larger set of stakeholders to set priorities and the sequencing of policy recommendations.

Contents

Tables

Summary

Dementia: A Looming Epidemic

Today, roughly 15 percent of Americans older than 70—an estimated 3.8 million people—are living with dementia.[1] By 2050, an estimated 13.8 million Americans age 65 and older will have Alzheimer's disease,[2] the most common form of dementia. Alzheimer's disease is the sixth leading cause of death in the United States and the fifth leading cause of death for those age 65 and older.[3] It is the only cause of death among the top ten in the United States for which there is no cure, no form of prevention, and no means of slowing its progression.[4] This public health burden increases when one considers the generally long duration of disability and dependence associated with the disease that requires long-term services and supports (LTSS). The burden of disease for Alzheimer's disease, measured by disability-adjusted life years, has also risen more than any other disease in the United States from 1990 to 2010.[5, 6]

Alzheimer's disease and related dementias are among the most costly of medical conditions. In 2013, a groundbreaking RAND study was the first to quantify the annual economic costs solely attributable to dementia in the United States.[1] The study estimated these costs at somewhere between $159 billion to $215 billion annually—sums that are similar to or greater than the costs attributable to heart disease or cancer. Moreover, these costs could more than double by 2040. The vast majority of costs associated with dementia among those 70 or older are attributable to LTSS rather than to medical services. Yet the LTSS system has typically not been well aligned with the needs of persons with dementia.

This report focuses on the LTSS system and its intersection with dementia care. Our purpose is to provide our recommendations for the highest-impact policy options. We also categorize them by the stakeholder groups that would have primary responsibility for implementing them to assist stakeholders in organizing a plan of action.

The Current State of Dementia LTSS

Service Delivery

LTSS can be provided by formal providers or informal caregivers. Informal care, which we refer to as family care, is unpaid care that is usually in the form of assistance from a relative or friend. The vast majority of LTSS—for all conditions, not just dementia—are provided by informal caregivers: as much as 80 percent, according to one estimate.[7] Although timely and accurate detection and diagnosis of dementia do not always occur within the scope of LTSS, they are critical for effective planning for dementia care and ensuring the quality of dementia care. However, unofficial estimates peg the proportion of those with dementia who are formally diagnosed at roughly half.[8–10] Furthermore, studies report that as few as half of those with dementia and their families receive support or guidance about its prognosis,[11, 12] and services available to them, following a diagnosis.[13, 14]

An important trend in the delivery of services by formal caregivers over the past 20 years has been a deliberate "rebalancing" of care away from such institutional settings as nursing homes and toward home- and community-based settings. This shift is reflected in the share of Medicaid spending for home- and community-based services (HCBS), which doubled between 1995 and 2011[15] and is growing at a much faster rate than spending on institutional services. However, it is uncertain how this trend specifically affects dementia care.

There are several critical gaps and challenges in LTSS service delivery. While the current LTSS landscape for dementia varies from state to state—largely because of differences in state Medicaid programs, which finance the majority of LTSS that are not paid for out of pocket—some general themes emerge on a national level.

As suggested above, detection and diagnosis remain problematic, and the use of biomarkers and other cognitive assessment tools, though showing signs of progress, remains in flux. The high cost of care also continues to pose a challenge. Publicly financed home- or community-based services provided by formal caregivers remain inaccessible for middle-income families because of Medicaid eligibility requirements. These middle-income families pay for these services out of pocket. The percentage of middle-class families that are expected to spend down their assets to Medicaid eligibility levels is projected to increase in the future, given the demographic changes stemming from the aging of the baby boomers and the dearth of family caregivers available to care for them.[16] Persons with dementia frequently experience transitions across the stages of dementia, including obtaining the initial diagnosis, advanced planning for financial concerns and health care considerations, driving cessation, managing behavioral symptoms, reduced decisionmaking capacity, changes in care settings, and preparing for the end of life. However, the settings and facilities that provide LTSS during these transitions frequently operate in silos with no overlap in or coordination across data systems.

Workforce

The dementia workforce is composed of both paid providers and family caregivers. More than 15 million Americans currently provide family care to family members or friends with dementia.[5] These informal caregivers, often referred to as family caregivers,[17] typically shoulder a heavy burden: nearly 40 percent reported quitting jobs or reducing work hours to care for a family member with dementia.[18] Many of these caregivers also experience negative physical and mental health effects.[18] Women in particular are more likely than men to suffer negative employment and health consequences.[19] Moreover, family caregivers frequently report that they are inadequately educated about the trajectory of dementia and community resources after a dementia diagnosis has been made.[20, 21]

Demographic trends suggest that the current heavy reliance on family caregiving is unsustainable. As the median age of the U.S. population, including baby boomers, trends upward, there will be a growing imbalance between the number of people needing care and family caregivers available to deliver it. To illustrate, the AARP Public Policy Institute estimates that the ratio of caregivers aged 45–64 to each person aged 80 and older who needs LTSS will decline from 7:1 in 2010 to less than 3:1 in 2050.[16]

With respect to formal care, the majority of those who provide LTSS are direct care workers, including nursing aides, home health aides, and personal- or home-care aides.[2] Inadequate training for dementia in the direct care workforce has been identified as a main contributor to poor quality of life, poor quality of care, abuse, and neglect in nursing homes.[22, 23] This workforce would benefit substantially from training in how to manage behavioral symptoms related to dementia.

Initiatives under way to improve training in dementia and elder care are a first step toward addressing this need.[24, 25] Another significant gap in the LTSS workforce stems from the growing imbalance between the demand for—and supply of—qualified, paid workers. This shortage results from high turnover and difficulty attracting qualified workers. Shortfalls in this workforce are often filled via the "gray market," meaning that untrained, low-cost caregivers are hired, leaving older adults vulnerable to poor or unregulated care. Compounding this problem: Certification requirements for paraprofessional caregivers are low to nonexistent in most states, and federal requirements are minimal (less than two weeks of training).

Financing

The costs of long-term paid caregiving for persons with dementia are high, and they increase sharply as cognitive impairment worsens. According to RAND estimates, the expense for home care borne by families (valued in terms of the replacement cost if such care was purchased in the home care market) accounts for approximately 50 percent of the costs of dementia care.[1] Furthermore, this estimate excludes economic costs associated with the caregiver's emotional well-being, health status, work productivity, foregone leisure activities, and increased risk of injury or death.

With respect to paid LTSS, Medicaid is the largest payer. Medicaid can cover nursing home care and paid care provided in the home or community, as well as assistance with personal care. In contrast, Medicare finances only hospice costs and a portion of short-stay, post-acute care for Medicare beneficiaries.[7, 16, 26, 27] However, Medicaid eligibility rules in many states require that individuals have assets no greater than $2,000. This restriction results in significant gaps in risk protection from high LTSS costs. People with adequate resources who plan early enough turn to private long-term care (LTC) insurance or out-of-pocket resources for financing, while lower-income individuals are covered through Medicaid, leaving the middle-income population at greatest risk for significant and possibly catastrophic LTSS cost with no readily available resources to finance their long-term dementia care. Inadequate personal savings for LTSS may increase the proportion of the population that risk impoverishing themselves and depending on Medicaid coverage. Programs to address this gap—such as the LTC State Partnership Program, currently available in 31 states to promote the purchase of private LTC coverage—did not increase the uptake of LTC coverage as much as expected,[28] and private insurance companies continue to struggle to get individuals to buy private LTC policies. At the same time, the costs of LTC policies continue to rise. In 2013, the federal Commission on Long-Term Care outlined several alternative mechanisms to address financing for LTSS but failed to reach consensus about the best financing approach. The Bipartisan Policy Center currently has an initiative to develop a plan for a sustainable means of financing and delivering LTSS and will issue policy recommendations in late 2014 for all LTSS, regardless of disease or condition.

Policy Options at the Intersection of LTSS and Dementia

Approach

We first reviewed four publicly available national plans and reports for strengthening LTSS and dementia care. All of these plans and reports have outlined strategies either for dementia[29–31] or for LTSS,[32, 33] but none have focused exclusively on their interrelationship. In addition, many of the strategies apply a top-down approach in which federal agencies are mainly held responsible for implementing the strategies. In our approach, we identified options through engagement with a range of stakeholders from federal, state, and local levels, including patients, the public, purchasers, formal and family providers, public and private payers, policymakers, and researchers. This approach is necessary to involve stakeholders in a continuous process to more effectively move policy forward. The result was a list of 38 priority policy options grouped into three categories: service delivery, workforce, and financing. This three-domain framework is the same used by the Commission on Long-Term Care.

To qualitatively determine which of the 38 dementia LTSS policy options were the most promising, we evaluated these 38 options against 14 impact, equity, and feasibility criteria and summarized their impact (high or low), their feasibility (high or low), and the stakeholders responsible for or affected by the policy option.

Priority Policy Options

We recommend that the 25 highest-impact policy options (Table S.1) should be considered for implementation immediately. Although our evaluation resulted in 25 priority policy options, many options cannot be pursued in isolation from others and must be bundled to optimize successful implementation and maximum impact on access, quality, and utilization of LTSS. One exception in which options conflict with each other and cannot be undertaken simultaneously is the two national LTSS financing system options to either create a national, voluntary opt-out public-private partnership insurance program or to adopt a national single-payer insurance system. In this case, both options were deemed as having high impact on dementia LTSS, but more research is needed to understand which of the two priority options is most feasible, for example, from a political standpoint. The 25 high-impact policy options are organized into five objectives:

- Increase public awareness of dementia to reduce stigma and promote earlier detection of signs and symptoms.
- Improve access to and utilization of LTSS for persons with dementia.
- Promote high-quality, person- and family caregiver–centered care.
- Provide better support for family caregivers of people with dementia.
- Reduce the burden of dementia LTSS costs on individuals and families.

Meeting each objective requires efforts across multiple sectors and by numerous stakeholders. Thus, we determined the primary stakeholders responsible for implementing these policy options. In addition, we used the same framework as the Commission on Long-Term Care and indicated which of the three domains each of the policy options falls under: service delivery, workforce, or financing.

Implementation of Policy Options

The stakeholders who are primarily responsible for carrying out the 25 priority policy options are providers, payers, and policymakers. Nonetheless, it is important to engage all stakeholders who play a supportive role or who would be affected by implementation. Patients and providers are among the stakeholders most likely to be affected by new policy, and they should therefore be engaged even when not designated to implement a policy. Cross-sector leadership for implementation can occur through multi-stakeholder conventions, multi-actor plans, and clear assignments of roles and responsibilities for implementation that maximize efficiency to overcome the silos that public and private payers; multiple government agencies; and multiple private, professional, and civic actors sometimes operate within.

Table S.1
25 High-Impact Policy Options for Dementia LTSS

Policy Option	Primary Stakeholders Responsible	Domain
Objective 1: Increase public awareness of dementia to reduce stigma and promote earlier detection of signs and symptoms.		
Create specialized and targeted outreach and education programs for the public, caregivers, professional services organizations, and persons with younger-onset dementia.	Providers—formal Policymakers—fed, st, loc	SD
Encourage providers' use of cognitive assessment tools for early dementia detection and recognition.	Providers—formal Policymakers—fed, st, loc Principal investigators	SD
Objective 2: Improve access to and utilization of LTSS for persons with dementia.		
Establish new and expand existing home- and community-based services (HCBS).	Providers—formal Policymakers—fed, st	SD
Integrate web- and other technology-based services into dementia LTSS.	Providers—formal Policymakers—fed, st Product makers	SD
Create new and improve existing incentives for the direct care workforce.	Providers—formal Policymakers—fed, st, loc	W
Expand nurse delegation laws in all states.	Policymakers—fed, st	W
Broaden Medicaid HCBS waiver programs, self-directed services, and states' infrastructures.	Payers—public Policymakers—fed, st	F
Include HCBS and managed care in state Medicaid plans.	Payers—public Policymakers—st	F
Refine Medicare post-acute care and hospice benefits.	Payers—public Policymakers—fed	F
Objective 3: Promote high-quality, person- and family caregiver–centered care.		
Establish Centers of Excellence models for dementia residential care through the end of life.	Providers—formal Payers—public, private Policymakers—fed	SD
Minimize transitions and improve coordination of care across providers, settings, and stages of dementia.	Providers—formal Policymakers—fed, st	SD
Expand financial incentives for bundled home, community, and institutional services.	Providers—formal Payers—public, private Policymakers—fed, st	SD
Establish cross-setting teams for persons with dementia, focused on returning the person to the community.	Providers—formal, family Payers—public, private Policymakers—fed, st	SD
Encourage the use of quality measurement to ensure consistent use of assessment tools for persons with dementia and their family caregivers.	Providers—formal Payers—public, private Policymakers—fed, st	SD

Table S.1—continued

Policy Option	Primary Stakeholders Responsible	Domain
Identify persons with dementia jointly with their family caregivers during emergent, acute, and post-acute care.	Providers—formal Product makers	SD
Standardize complementary assessment tools for persons with dementia and their family caregivers.	Providers—formal Policymakers—fed, st Principal investigators	SD
Create new and disseminate existing dementia best practices and training programs for professional and paraprofessional care workers.	Providers—formal Policymakers—fed, st, loc	W
Provide specialized geriatric training to direct care professionals while in school.	Providers—formal Policymakers—fed, st, loc	W
Objective 4: Provide better support for family caregivers of people with dementia.		
Provide dementia-specific training and information about resources to family caregivers and volunteer groups.	Providers—formal	W
Offer business and individual tax incentives to promote family caregiving.	Policymakers—fed, st, loc	W
Expand financial compensation programs to family caregivers.	Payers—public, private Policymakers—fed, st	W
Expand family-friendly workplace policies.	Purchasers Policymakers—fed, st, loc	W
Objective 5: Reduce the burden of dementia LTSS costs on individuals and families.		
Link private LTC insurance to health insurance.	Payers—public, private	F
Create a national, voluntary opt-out LTC insurance program through a public-private partnership.	Payers—public, private Policymakers—fed, st	F
Adopt a national single-payer LTC insurance system.	Payers—public Policymakers—fed	F

NOTES: fed = federal, st = state, loc = local, SD = service delivery, W = workforce, and F = financing. Family caregivers are defined broadly and include informal caregivers who are relatives, partners, friends, or neighbors who have a significant relationship with, and who provide a broad range of assistance for, an older adult or an adult with chronic or disabling conditions.[17] Principal investigators include researchers and research funders.

Although some of these options are rated high for potential impact, they may face significant barriers to implementation. In some cases, the barriers are legal in nature. Existing legislation may need to be modified or removed, or new legislation may be needed to authorize the policy, as in the proposed expansion of HCBS programs. Barriers may also be operational, as in the proposed links between LTC insurance and health insurance products. Or barriers may be political, as in the expected opposition by some parties to a single-payer LTC insurance system or to a voluntary opt-out public-private partnership insurance program. Barriers to implementation, however, can change quickly, and every effort should be made to reduce or eliminate them.

Priority Research Directions

The primary objective of this report was to identify and evaluate policy options. As a byproduct of our stakeholder discussions, five priorities for future research were also identified. These research options represent stakeholders' perceptions of the most urgent research priorities and are only a subset of a longer list of research directions that should be undertaken to support the implementation of policy options outlined in this blueprint. Stakeholders suggested research investment in the following areas:

- applied research programs on the delivery of dementia LTSS
- costs and quality of dementia care provided through nurse delegation programs
- LTSS financing solutions for the federal government and persons with dementia
- impact of Medicare reforms on dementia care
- uptake of private LTC insurance and consumer understanding of Health Insurance Portability and Accountability Act (HIPAA) tax incentives.

Comparison of the RAND Blueprint with Other Dementia or Long-Term Services and Supports National Plans and Reports

Stakeholders identified ten policy options unique to our report that did not appear in the National Plan or the three national reports. These ten unique policy options generally focused on topics that highlight challenges that may be exacerbated for dementia, including its progressive nature, the presence of difficult-to-manage behavioral symptoms, the strong dependence on family caregivers for support, and the need for financial planning because of high LTSS costs. Our findings suggest that the 25 priority policy options for dementia LTSS are in line with and further support the broader LTSS recommendations made by the Commission on Long-Term Care.[32, 33] Nevertheless, as the numbers of the U.S. older adult population and the numbers of those with dementia swell, these ten unique policy options may also be important to turn to in the near term.

Conclusion: A Blueprint for LTSS Through the Lens of Dementia Care

This blueprint provides 25 priority policy options that address challenges with (1) stigma and early detection of signs and symptoms of dementia that can affect downstream access to care and quality of care; (2) inadequate access to—and measurement of—quality LTSS; (3) fragmented delivery systems that may affect persons with dementia more severely because of the heavy reliance on services both outside and inside the traditional health care system and on family caregivers; (4) insufficient resource-finding infrastructure, employer programs, and financial resources to support family caregivers of people with dementia; and (5) insufficient public and private options to help individuals and their families deal with the potentially crushing costs associated with dementia LTSS.

Dementia presents distinctive issues within the LTSS system because of its high prevalence, progressive nature, effects on behavior and ability to self-manage care due to impaired cognitive and decisionmaking capabilities, frequency of care transitions, risk of elder abuse, high rate of comorbid health conditions, heavy reliance and resulting health impacts on caregivers, and higher costs associated with LTSS compared to other chronic conditions in late life.

The strengths of our study include the engagement of interviewees representing stakeholder perspectives from across the health care system, the evaluation of policy options across 14 criteria, and the prioritization and comparison of policy options with options recommended by other national efforts. More importantly, this is the only evaluation that places a spotlight on policy options in LTSS for dementia specifically. Despite these strengths, we note several limitations.

Future work should include convening a larger group of stakeholders to assign low, moderate, or high strength-of-evidence metrics to each of the 14 impact, feasibility, and equity ratings and to build consensus on how best to select and carry out priority policy options. This larger sample of stakeholders should consider whether policy options could have varied results depending on the types of dementia. Future research should also undertake a stakeholder-engaged process to prioritize research needs, much like those conducted previously for LTSS research.[34] The qualitative rating approach we used should be supplemented by conducting systematic literature reviews of evidence-based programs, analyses of each policy option's cost-effectiveness, and analyses using existing administrative and clinical data. These types of studies would facilitate a better understanding of the strength of evidence for each rating and relative importance of policies in terms of allocation of resources and urgency of implementation.

In the process of consensus-building, we recommend that dementia LTSS stakeholders work together to develop metrics—key performance indicators of LTSS system performance for persons affected by dementia—in order to monitor progressive improvements on each of the five overarching objectives. Examples of metrics may include

- a target percentage of the estimated population with dementia that has received a diagnosis
- a target percentage of the Medicaid-eligible diagnosed population that has a quality care plan and is receiving desired HCBS
- cross-setting teams and person-centered care plans for a target percentage of persons with diagnosed dementia
- dementia-specific training received by a target proportion of family caregivers within a specific time frame following a diagnosis
- a target percentage reduction in median out-of-pocket dementia LTSS costs for persons with dementia and their families.

Process metrics may also be measured, including the extent of communication between stakeholders, the number of panel roundtable discussions that take place, the amount of research funding allocated to determine data sources, the establishment of monitoring plans for meeting metrics, and the adoption of responsibility for taking action on metrics by stakeholders across multiple sectors.

In conclusion, it is our hope that this research will highlight the need for stakeholders to focus on dementia LTSS policies and will serve as the foundation for a larger group of stakeholders to build consensus around the dementia LTSS policy options that should be pursued most urgently.

Acknowledgments

We wish to thank several individuals who contributed to this report. Charles J. Zwick provided the philanthropic support to carry out this research, and we thank him for his continued support to help RAND research achieve maximum impact. We also express gratitude to our RAND research support team, including Craig Matsuda, David M. Adamson, Stacy Fitzsimmons, and Shawna Beck-Sullivan, for their help over the course of the project and with preparing this report.

The research presented herein relied on key informant interviews with a diverse group of stakeholders who are nationally recognized experts and representatives of national, state, and local organizations. We thank this report's advisors and interviewees for volunteering their time and providing invaluable contributions to the development of this report. Individuals who consented to being acknowledged, whether they were interviewees or advisors, include

Gretchen E. Alkema (The SCAN Foundation)
Jim Beck (Home Instead Senior Care)
Lawrence Becker (Xerox Corporation)
Maribeth Bersani (Assisted Living Federation of America)
Richard Birkel (National Council on Aging)
Debra L. Cherry (Alzheimer's Association, California Southland Chapter)
Marc A. Cohen (LifePlans, Inc.)
Jennifer Dexter (Easter Seals)
Charlotte Eliopoulos (American Association for Long Term Care Nursing)
Lynn Friss Feinberg (AARP Public Policy Institute)
Charles J. Fuschillo, Jr. (Alzheimer's Foundation of America)
Richard P. Grimes (Assisted Living Federation of America)
Mark Hensley (North Carolina Department of Health and Human Services)
Drew Holzapfel (Global CEO Initiative on Alzheimer's Disease)
Gail Gibson Hunt (National Alliance for Caregiving)
Marianne Hurley (Warren Alpert Medicine School of Brown University)
Ian Kremer (Leaders Engaged on Alzheimer's Disease [LEAD] Coalition)
MaryAnne Lindeblad (Washington State Health Care Authority)

William L. Minnix (LeadingAge)
Corrinne Altman Moore (MassHealth)
Linda Netterville (Meals on Wheels Association of America)
Lisa R. Shugarman (The SCAN Foundation)
Lorie Van Tilburg (Southern Caregiver Resource Center)
George Vradenburg (USAgainstAlzheimer's)
Andrew R. Hoehn (RAND)
Jeffrey Wasserman (RAND)
Krishna B. Kumar (RAND)
Michael D. Hurd (RAND)
David M. Adamson (RAND)
Craig Matsuda (RAND)
Linda G. Martin (RAND)

Our report benefited from astute guidance provided by a four-member Advisory Council consisting of RAND Health Advisory Board members. We thank Pedro José Greer, Jr. (Florida International University Herbert Wertheim College of Medicine), Susan Hullin (Arrowwood Partners, LLC), Mary Naylor (University of Pennsylvania School of Nursing), and Bradley Perkins (Human Longevity, Inc.) for their input over the course of the project.

Finally, we acknowledge Neil S. Wenger (RAND/UCLA) and Katie Maslow (Institute of Medicine), who provided invaluable advice and highly insightful comments in their quality assurance review of this report.

Abbreviations

ABLE Act	Achieving a Better Life Experience Act
AFA	Alzheimer's Foundation of America
CLASS	Community Living Assistance Services and Supports
HCBS	home- and community-based services
HIPAA	Health Insurance Portability and Accountability Act
LTC	long-term care
LTSS	long-term services and supports
NAPA	National Alzheimer's Project Act
POLST	Physician Orders for Life-Sustaining Treatment

CHAPTER ONE

Introduction

Statement of the Problem

Dementia is a debilitating and progressive condition that affects memory and cognitive functioning, results in behavioral and psychiatric disorders, and leads to decline in the ability to engage in activities of daily living and self-care.[35] In 2010, 14.7 percent of persons older than age 70 in the United States had dementia. With the expected doubling of the number of Americans age 65 or older from 40 million in 2010 to more than 88 million in 2050, the annual number of new dementia cases is also expected to double by 2050, barring any significant medical breakthroughs.[4]

Alzheimer's disease, which accounts for 60 to 80 percent of dementia cases, is the sixth leading cause of death in the United States overall and the fifth leading cause of death for those age 65 and older.[3] Additionally, recent research suggests that deaths attributable to Alzheimer's disease might be underreported such that it could be the third leading cause of death overall.[36] It is the only cause of death among the top ten in the United States without a way to prevent it, cure it, or even slow its progression.[4] In addition to Alzheimer's disease, some of the other common types of dementia and conditions that cause dementia include

- vascular dementia
- Lewy body dementia
- frontotemporal dementia
- Huntington's disease
- Parkinson's disease
- traumatic brain injury.

In 2013, Michael Hurd and colleagues at RAND published a landmark study on the monetary costs of dementia in the United States.[1] He and his colleagues estimated that the condition, with costs of $159 billion to $215 billion annually, takes a similar or greater economic toll on the nation than heart disease or cancer. The fiscal year 2014 bill summary of the Senate Committee on Appropriations noted that the total payments for health care, long-term services and supports (LTSS), and hospice for people with dementia are projected to increase from $203 billion in 2013 to $1.2 trillion in 2050. Costs for Medicare and Medicaid related to dementia are estimated to rise by 500 percent.

As the baby boomers age, the number of Americans who will need LTSS is expected to double by 2050.[38] This cohort is approaching the peak age of dementia onset. With more single-parent and single-child households, the fact that caregiving is most frequently provided by family caregivers raises the question of who will take care of the growing number of older adults who may develop dementia. In addition, life expectancies have increased so that it is possible for two generations within one family to be living with dementia at the same time.

The current acute and LTSS system is fragmented and costly to federal and state governments and to families who incur out-of-pocket costs not covered by public or private insurance. It is clear that current policies must be adapted to support the projected increase in the number of persons with dementia who will need LTSS in the coming decades.

Goals of the RAND Dementia LTSS Blueprint

Gaps in the LTSS system and dementia care overlap to a great extent. This blueprint identifies policy options that could be undertaken to address challenges at the intersection of LTSS and dementia. It also identifies the stakeholders who could take the lead on the implementation of these policy options. We interviewed a sample of stakeholders representing the larger population of dementia LTSS stakeholders and asked them two key questions:

1. What problems or challenges do they face in the delivery of care, development of policy, and research on LTSS for persons with dementia?
2. How can policy address those challenges?

We then outlined the policy options identified by stakeholders and evaluate those options on impact and feasibility of implementation. These evaluations informed our blueprint for the most impactful policy options for dementia LTSS stakeholders to undertake in the near term.

Our analyses serve as a foundation upon which to engage stakeholders in a larger debate and to conduct robust evaluations to build consensus on a set and sequencing of policy recommendations to pursue. While our goal was to outline priority policy options, individual policy options cannot be pursued in isolation from others. As such, we note which policy options could be bundled to optimize successful implementation and maximum impact on access, quality, and utilization of LTSS, even if a policy is not a priority policy option identified in our evaluation.

This blueprint is intended for use by policymakers, providers, researchers, advocates, caregivers, and persons with dementia. We have organized the blueprint around five main goals:

1. Identify gaps in dementia LTSS within three domains: service delivery, workforce, and financing.
2. Review national plans and reports on dementia or LTSS policy.
3. Identify policy options to address gaps in the LTSS system for persons with dementia, from the perspectives of a diverse array of stakeholders.
4. Conduct an independent evaluation of policy options.
5. Prioritize policy options by impact, feasibility, dementia stage, and stakeholder group.

Although the policy options outlined in this blueprint may not have broad application to other countries, a global agenda must be pursued, as the prevalence of dementia globally is expected to triple between 2013 and 2050,[39] while at the same time developing countries will experience increasing rates of female participation in the workforce, longer life expectancies, and diminishing family sizes, which may affect the LTSS systems in these countries. These movements toward a global agenda include efforts currently under way by the World Health Organization and the action steps following the U.K.-hosted Dementia Summit held in December 2013 to create a Global Fund and an interparliamentary group to tackle dementia. Cross-national performance assessments of dementia LTSS systems can also be developed that would measure systems' performance against metrics.

Why Focus on the Intersection of Dementia LTSS?

The vast majority of costs—between 75 percent and 84 percent—associated with dementia among those 70 and older are attributable to LTSS, rather than medical services.[1] Moreover, there are significant additional costs attributable to increased use of medical services by persons with dementia because of family caregivers' potential inability to manage behaviors, falls, and acute episodes related to comorbidities due to reduced self-management capabilities for persons with dementia.[40] LTSS include assistance with activities of daily living (e.g., bathing, dressing, eating, and walking), instrumental activities of daily living (e.g., meal preparation, medication management, transportation), and health maintenance for people with limitations because of physical, cognitive, chronic, or developmental conditions. Because the study by Hurd and colleagues found that a high proportion of dementia costs are related to nursing home care and formal and family home care, we contend that the most promising avenues for policy action with near-term benefits related to dementia involve focusing on the intersection between dementia and LTSS.

The current LTSS landscape suggests that there is considerable room for improvement in the system; more could be done to align the system with the needs of dementia patients and caregivers. Below we discuss challenges that are especially relevant for dementia care, as well as gaps in the current state of service delivery, workforce, and financing for dementia LTSS.

Caregiving for Persons with Dementia Is Especially Challenging

LTSS can be provided through informal and formal means. Informal care, which we refer to as family care, is defined as assistance from a relative, partner, friend, or neighbor who has a significant relationship with, and who provides a broad range of assistance for, an older adult or an adult with chronic or disabling conditions.[17] Formal care is provided by paid caregivers.

The magnitude of the challenges associated with dementia LTSS is large if one were to consider formal caregiving alone. Persons with dementia experience, on average, more care settings and more transitions between care settings than do older adults with other chronic conditions.[41] Regardless of health condition, these transitions, particularly those following hospital discharges, are periods of major risk of medical errors and infections, stress, and agitation that can lead to future hospital readmissions and delirium.[42, 43] Moreover, LTSS providers usually store data in systems that are not integrated, which can contribute to fragmentation of care, lack of coordination between services, and duplication of services.[44]

Most diseases and conditions that cause dementia are progressive, and there are currently no treatments to halt the progression of the condition or its symptoms. The hallmark symptoms of dementia are impaired cognition and function. As such, persons with dementia are less able to self-manage their typically multiple comorbidities. Persons with dementia have a greater reliance on family caregivers, and for a longer period of time, for assistance with activities of daily living when compared with older adults receiving care for other diseases.[45–48] As one indicator of the greater need for formal care among persons with dementia, 48.5 percent of nursing home residents and 30.1 percent of home health patients in 2012 had dementia.[7]

Over time, persons with dementia may experience further behavioral and functional declines, fail to recognize loved ones, lower their social filters, and become verbally and physically combative.[49] As a result, they may become more abusive and be abused themselves, increase their isolation, and rely more heavily on their caregivers. Recent research suggests that abuse is commonly experienced by people with dementia,[50] with approximately half of people with dementia having experienced some kind of verbal, physical, or psychological abuse or neglect from their caregivers.[51] Moreover, persons with dementia are thought to be at greater risk for abuse compared to older adults without dementia.[52] This may be due to their cognitive impairment, loss of ability to communicate challenges, and increased dependence on their caregivers.

Persons with dementia assessed in primary care settings have 2.4 chronic medical conditions on average,[53] and persons with dementia or cognitive impairment have more serious comorbidity than those without cognitive impairment.[46] Although there is little evidence to suggest that the number of comorbid conditions is different for persons with and without dementia,[53] it is possible that the inability to self-manage for comorbid conditions results in the higher costs observed for persons with dementia and comorbid conditions compared to those without dementia with the same comorbid conditions.[54] This might also explain why community-dwelling elderly Medicare beneficiaries with dementia were more likely than others to be hospitalized and visit the emergency department in a given year, both overall and also for potentially avoidable conditions.[55] LTSS needs for persons with dementia evolve toward ever-greater intensity of care, and they typically experience more transitions in care than those without a dementia diagnosis,[41] from family care settings to formal home- and community-based services (HCBS) to institutional care, as well as from acute care to skilled nursing care to institutional care or HCBS. Coexisting medical conditions influence where a person with dementia is likely to receive the best care,[56] the kinds of help he or she needs from family and formal caregivers, the costs of care,[54] and, therefore, the kinds of training and support those caregivers need to provide high-quality care.

Vulnerable Populations Are at Risk for Dementia and Inadequate LTSS Coverage

Persons with a family history of dementia, racial/ethnic minorities, and individuals with lower education and incomes are more likely to be diagnosed with dementia.[57–59] Lower-income individuals are also less likely to be able to pay for private long-term care insurance or formal HCBS.

Individuals with Down syndrome represent another vulnerable population. Studies suggest that more than 75 percent of those with Down syndrome age 65 and older have Alzheimer's disease, which is nearly six times higher than the disease's rate among those age 65 and older who do not have Down syndrome.[60] Individuals with Down syndrome usually have formal LTSS coverage through Medicaid. However, any reliance on parent caregivers becomes more challenging as individuals with Down syndrome and their parents age.

Individuals with younger-onset dementia (onset before age 65) may not receive accurate diagnoses, are not covered by Medicare without an eligible disability, may be at greater risk for early departure from the workforce, and are at risk for loss of employer-sponsored health insurance. These patients may therefore be considered an especially vulnerable population.

Persons with advanced dementia, greater severity and longer duration of symptoms, and lower responsiveness to interventions are also at risk for inadequate LTSS coverage. Measures of symptom heterogeneity and heterogeneity of treatment effects might therefore also be considered important indicators of vulnerability.

The LTSS Delivery System Is Fragmented, and Quality of Care Is Variable

LTSS can be provided by formal providers or informal caregivers. Informal care, which we refer to as family care, usually means unpaid assistance from a relative or friend. The vast majority of LTSS—for all conditions, not just dementia—are provided by informal caregivers: as much as 80 percent, according to one estimate.[7] Though detection and diagnosis do not always occur within the scope of LTSS, they are critical to planning for dementia care, especially for those in the early stages of dementia. Yet, although there is no figure for the proportion of those with dementia who are formally diagnosed, informal calculations estimate the proportion at roughly half.[8, 9, 10] Furthermore, studies report that few individuals with a dementia diagnosis and their families receive support or guidance about its prognosis,[11, 14] its trajectory, and community resources following a diagnosis.[13, 20, 61] Although federal mandates exist for the measurement of nursing home care, poor quality and weak federal oversight remain major problems.

An important trend in the delivery of services by formal caregivers over the past 20 years has been a deliberate "rebalancing" of care away from such institutional settings as nursing homes and toward HCBS. This shift is reflected in the share of Medicaid spending for HCBS, which doubled between 1995 and 2011[15] and is growing at a much faster rate than spending on institutional services. However, it is uncertain how this trend specifically affects dementia care because there are no measures for quality of care, such as improvement in rates of post-diagnostic care, LTSS resource availability and utilization, and care outcomes.

There are several critical gaps and challenges in LTSS service delivery. As noted, detection and diagnosis remain problematic, and the use of biomarkers and other assessment tools, though showing signs of progress, remains in flux. The high cost of care also continues to pose a barrier to accessing the LTSS system. Formal home- or community-based care and institutional care remain inaccessible for middle-income families due either to Medicaid requirements, which restrict eligibility to those with assets below $2,000, or to the high cost of private LTC insurance.[18] Finally, system fragmentation and a lack of coordinated care across settings pose challenges.[44, 62, 63] Research has shown that involving caregivers in care decisions and transitions is critical to promoting high-quality care and avoiding adverse events.[64] However, this does not occur systematically because primary care, ambulatory care, emergency care, acute care, post-acute care, and community and institutional LTSS facilities and providers typically operate in silos with no overlap in data systems.

The Dementia LTSS Workforce Is Insufficiently Staffed, Trained, and Supported

Most of the burden of caring for people with dementia is shouldered by family and friends. More than 15 million Americans currently provide family care to relatives or friends with dementia.[5] These family caregivers[17] typically shoulder a heavy burden: Nearly 40 percent reported quitting jobs or reducing work hours to care for a family member with dementia.[18] Many of these caregivers also experience negative physical and mental health effects. Sixty-five percent of family caregivers are female,[65] and female caregivers are more likely than male caregivers to suffer negative employment and health consequences.[19] Family caregivers may also find themselves dealing with a range of behavioral challenges that are more common to dementia than to other chronic conditions in late life: wandering, incontinence, agitation, paranoia, repetitive speech, sleeplessness, poor hygiene, outbursts and sexually inappropriate actions, hallucinations, and shadowing or following others around.[66]

Caregivers who care for family members with dementia, on average, experience more stress, give up their vacations or hobbies more often, have less time for other family members, and report more work-related difficulties than those who care for persons with other physical impairments.[67, 68] They also experience higher rates of anxiety and depression,[69, 70] higher rates of utilization of clinical and acute care services,[71] and, in some cases, higher risk of mortality.[72, 73] Caregivers of family members with dementia spent more hours per day providing care compared to caregivers of persons without dementia, and even compared to persons with cognitive impairment that is not dementia.[70] As symptoms of dementia progress, the need for care and supports for caregivers may intensify; persons with dementia generally receive more care from family members and other unpaid caregivers as the condition progresses.[5] While interventions exist to help reduce the negative aspects of dementia family caregiving, their effects on caregivers and the care recipients are variable, and it is unclear whether there are any differences in the effects of these interventions by clinical, racial/ethnic, and socioeconomic characteristics.[5, 74]

With respect to formal care, about 70–80 percent of those who provide LTSS are direct care workers,[75] including nursing aides, home health aides, and home- or personal-care aides. This workforce benefits substantially from training in how to manage behavioral symptoms related to dementia. Inadequate training for dementia in the direct care workforce has been identified as a main contributor to poor quality of care, abuse, and neglect in nursing homes.[76] Another significant gap in the LTSS workforce stems from the growing imbalance between the demand for—and supply of—qualified paid workers.[33,77] This shortage results from high turnover and difficulty attracting qualified workers. Shortfalls in this workforce are often filled via the "gray market," meaning that untrained, low-cost caregivers are hired, leaving older adults vulnerable to poor or unregulated quality of care.[78]

Over the longer term, shortages in both the paid and unpaid workforces are expected to worsen. Demographic trends suggest that the heavy reliance on family caregiving in particular is unsustainable. As the median age of the U.S. population trends upward and family sizes shrink, there will be a growing imbalance between the number of people needing care and those available to deliver it.[16]

LTSS Are Expensive, and Financing Mechanisms Are Inadequate for Many Families

The costs of long-term caregiving for persons with dementia are high, and they increase sharply as cognitive impairment worsens. According to RAND estimates, the expense for home care borne by families (valued in terms of the replacement cost if such care was purchased in the home care market) accounts for approximately 50 percent of the costs of dementia care.[1] Furthermore, this estimate excludes economic costs associated with the caregiver's emotional well-being, work productivity, foregone leisure activities, and increased risk of death.

With respect to paid LTSS, Medicaid is the largest single payer.[32, 79] Medicaid can cover nursing home care and paid care provided in the home or community, as well as assistance with personal care, for very–low-income segments of the population. By contrast, Medicare finances only hospice costs and a portion of short-stay, post-acute care for Medicare beneficiaries.[7, 26, 27] The Alzheimer's Association[5, 80] has estimated that the average per-person Medicaid spending for Medicare beneficiaries age 65 and older with dementia is 19 times higher than the average per-person Medicaid spending for comparable Medicare beneficiaries without dementia.

However, Medicaid eligibility rules in many states require that individuals have assets no greater than $2,000, and this restriction results in significant gaps in financing. People with adequate resources who plan early enough turn to private LTC insurance for financing, while lower-income individuals are covered through Medicaid, leaving a vast middle-income population with no viable options for financing long-term dementia care other than spending their savings. Given often inadequate levels of retirement savings, this may result in widespread impoverishment in the coming years. Programs to address this gap—such as the LTC State Partnership Program, currently available in 31 states to promote the purchase of private LTC coverage—have not substantially increased the uptake of LTC coverage,[28] and private insurance companies continue to struggle to get individuals to buy private LTC policies. At the same time, the costs of LTC policies continue to rise. In 2013, the federal Commission on Long-Term Care outlined several steps to address financing for LTSS, but it failed to reach consensus about the best financing approach. The Bipartisan Policy Center currently has an initiative to recommend a sustainable means of financing and delivering LTSS, and it will issue policy recommendations in late 2014.

RAND's Blueprint Builds on Current U.S. Dementia or LTSS Strategies
National Dementia Plans

In response to aging trends in the United States, combined with the growing dementia epidemic, the National Alzheimer's Project Act (NAPA) was signed into law in January 2011. NAPA called for a national plan for dementia, and in May 2012, the first *National Plan to Address Alzheimer's Disease* (National Plan)[81] was published. We reviewed this 2012 National Plan, the 2013 update to the 2012 National Plan,[82] and the Alzheimer's Foundation of America's (AFA) 2012 *Time to Build* report.[31] The National Plan provides a solid strategy to address dementia care needs in the United States. Although the plan has five goals, federal investment allocated within NAPA is most heavily focused on improvement for prevention and treatment research rather than on improvement in care and support. Improvements to the quality, access, availability, and affordability of LTSS are needed to address current and ongoing needs of the 5.2 million Americans currently afflicted with Alzheimer's disease, which account for 60–80 percent of dementia cases, and 15 million family caregivers.[5] An overview of the National Plan and a comparison of the National Plan and the AFA report are presented in Appendix B (Tables B.2–B.6). The appendixes to this report are available for PDF download at www.rand.org/t/RR597 under the download tab.

National LTSS Plans

In 2010, the federal government tried to boost long-term care for the aging with the Community Living Assistance Services and Supports (CLASS) Act. The act proposed a voluntary, opt-out long-term care insurance program. However, because the administration deemed it too difficult to implement and financially unsustainable, the provision was repealed as part of the American Taxpayer Relief Act.[83–85] Following the dissolution of the CLASS Act, a bipartisan, 15-member federal Commission on Long-Term Care outlined a plan for LTSS in September 2013, containing 28 specific recommendations in the domains of service delivery, workforce, and financing.[32] In addition, an alternative report was issued by five members of the Commission on Long-Term Care[33] regarding finance issues. A comparison of these LTSS reports is presented in Appendix B (Tables B.7–B.9; the appendixes are available at www.rand.org/t/RR597 under the download tab).

State Dementia Plans

Although national plans and policies provide guidance and structure on how to improve dementia LTSS, the implementation of such policies often occurs at the state or local level. As of March 2014, 36 states have dementia plans, and 7 states are in the process of developing plans.[86] Most of the state plans outline goals and recommendations, and many provide information about local resources. The Alzheimer's Association reviewed state dementia plans that were available in 2012 and provided a side-by-side comparison of state plans by domain.[87] We summarize the 2012 Alzheimer's Association comparison of LTSS-related recommendations in Appendix B (Table B.10; the appendixes are available at www.rand.org/t/RR597 under the download tab). Overall, state dementia plans address the LTSS domains of public awareness, early detection and diagnosis, care and case management, quality of care, health care system capacity, training, workforce development, HCBS, long-term care, caregivers, research, brain health, data collection, safety, legal issues, and state government structure. However, state dementia plans vary in the domains they cover and in the level of detail provided within each domain. States also differ in their current stage of implementation, and there is substantial variability in the capacity and quality for LTSS across states.[88]

The majority of formal LTSS for low-income populations are paid for by Medicaid, and state Medicaid staff provide the front-line interaction with beneficiaries. State insurance commissions regulate the private LTC insurance market, which is currently the only LTC insurance option for individuals who are not eligible for Medicaid. States with innovative dementia care programs and policies often provide evidence to support the scaling-up of such programs to a national level. While states play an important role in care innovation, clinical translation, and implementation of evidence-based research programs for the service delivery, workforce, and financing of dementia LTSS, blueprints such as this document can serve as guidance for policymakers at various levels, as well as functioning as a motivating force for federal dollars to be allocated to states in order to build capacity to administer front-line LTSS to state residents. For example, the Healthy Brain Initiative and its road map series have provided guidance on how national and state partnerships along with local aging services can connect and collaborate in order to address cognitive health.[89]

RAND's Blueprint Focuses on U.S. Dementia LTSS

While there is overlap between current dementia plans and LTSS policy recommendations, only the NAPA process emphasized the intersection between dementia and LTSS. In our view, however, NAPA did not not adequately define a comprehensive, multisector implementation pathway for its policy recommendations. The importance of this intersection is apparent, given the growing dementia epidemic and the need for focused policies and programs to address the LTSS issues for persons with dementia and their caregivers and the high costs of dementia, particularly out-of-pocket LTSS costs. To our knowledge, no national plan to date has focused on multisector strategies specifically for dementia LTSS.

Most strategies to date outline policy recommendations for which mainly federal and sometimes state agencies are held responsible for implementing strategies. By contrast, our goal was to create a blueprint that was driven not only by federal policymakers, but that also incorporates the priority challenges and policy options identified by state and local public and private stakeholders, including patients, providers, purchasers, payers, policymakers, and researchers. This stakeholder-engaged approach is also necessary to involve stakeholders in a continuous process to move policy forward. Indeed, the World Health Organization's strategy document *Dementia: A Public Health Priority*[8] notes that involving stakeholders in a collaborative process to identify issues that are important to them is key, stating, "sustained action and coordination is required across multiple levels and with all stakeholders—at international, national, regional and local levels."

Organization of the Report

This report contains three chapters. Chapter Two presents the dementia LTSS policy options that we identified through our stakeholder engagement process, and our mapping of these policy options against existing action steps recommended by national plans and reports on either dementia or LTSS. Chapter Three reports on RAND's evaluation of those policy options and prioritization of policy options by impact, feasibility, stage of dementia, and stakeholder group. We conclude Chapter Three with our recommendations for a blueprint to improve dementia LTSS in the United States.

A separate document titled *Improving Dementia Long-Term Care: Appendixes* (the appendixes are available at www.rand.org/t/RR597 under the download tab) provides a more detailed description of the current state of LTSS service delivery, workforce, and financing; a summary of prior dementia or long-term care plans and reports; the landscape of current action steps in existing plans or reports on either LTSS or dementia; detailed methods for the stakeholder-led identification of policy options; full descriptions of the policy options; RAND's evaluation of those policy options against 14 criteria; and our organization of the policy options by stakeholder group and stages of dementia.

CHAPTER TWO

Stakeholder-Engaged Policy Identification

Overview

As described in the previous chapter, this blueprint is meant to jointly address long-term care and dementia policy challenges and solutions. As such, a key goal was to gather insight from individuals with a variety of perspectives about the challenges associated with delivering LTSS for persons with dementia and to identify policy options that could address those challenges.

In this chapter, we present the methods and results of RAND's stakeholder-engaged policy identification process. We first provide a brief overview of our stakeholder identification and interview methods. The remaining sections present the 38 policy options that were identified by stakeholders during interviews, as well as a brief comparison of the policy options with recommendations made in other reports.

Methods for Identifying and Evaluating Policy Options

We adopted a recently developed taxonomy known as the 7Ps framework[90] to identify 30 interviewees. (See Appendix C for more details; the appendixes are available at www.rand.org/t/RR597 under the download tab.) Table 2.1 presents general descriptions of the interviewees and the stakeholder categories they represented. In this report, family caregivers are identified as patients when services are delivered to a family caregiver. Alternatively, family caregivers are identified as providers when LTSS are delivered by a family caregiver.

We conducted structured interviews by telephone around two key questions:

1. What problems or challenges do you face in the delivery of care, development of policy, or research on LTSS for persons with dementia?
2. How can policy address the problems or challenges you identified?

Data from each interview were independently extracted by two research staff and adjudicated in conference. Initially, 184 policy options were identified. After assigning thematic codes to each of the options,[91] we combined and synthesized similar policy options by thematic code, until the smallest number of policy options was identified without altering the meaning and intentions of the policy options. We arrived at a final list of 38 policy options.

Table 2.1
Summary of Stakeholders Interviewed

Category	Types	N
Patients and public	Patients, patient advocates, family caregivers	7
Providers	Formal and family caregivers, LTSS providers	8
Purchasers	Public and private employers	2
Payers	Private insurers, Medicare, Medicaid	4
Policymakers	Federal and state regulators, associations	5
Product makers	Drug, device, and health information technology manufacturers	0
Principal investigators	Health and human services, aging, and dementia policy researchers and research funders	4
TOTAL		30

We present these 38 stakeholder-identified policy options in their entirety. That is, we report the options without applying any preconceived presumptions about the existence or magnitude of the problems identified. We note that we reported the policy options as stated by the stakeholders, and we did not confirm, via systematic reviews of evidence-based practices or original data analyses, that the policy option that was suggested as a solution to a challenge was in fact the correct solution. We present these policy options to serve as the foundation for ongoing deliberations to assess the correctness, relative importance, and timeliness of each challenge and policy option.

To evaluate the policy options, we applied 14 criteria, described in Table 2.2, that were grouped into three domains: impact, equity, and feasibility. The methods for selecting these evaluation criteria are provided in Appendix C (the appendixes are available at www.rand.org/t/RR597 under the download tab). Two RAND reviewers independently evaluated the 38 policy options by applying stoplight ratings for each policy option against the 14 criteria. Stoplight ratings include a green indicator for policy options that achieve their desired effect, yellow for options achieving a neutral effect, red for options achieving an undesired effect, and gray for an undetermined effect. Reviewers' stoplight ratings were compared, and differences were adjudicated in conference. Appendix C presents detailed methods for identifying and evaluating the policy options.

Stakeholder-Identified Policy Options

The 38 policy options identified by our stakeholders are presented in Tables 2.3, 2.4, and 2.5 and are grouped into the same three categories used by the Commission on Long-Term Care: service delivery, workforce, and financing.[32] In the description column, we indicate policy options that may be grouped together and those

Table 2.2
RAND Evaluation Criteria

Dimension		Criterion	Description
Impact	Access	Awareness	Patient and caregiver knowledge of needs and available services
		Availability	Capacity of local services and resources
		Utilization	Use of services and resources
	Quality	Effectiveness	Delivery of services that improve patient and caregiver outcomes
		Safety	Avoidance of injuries
		Coordination of care	Care integration across dementia stages and settings
		Patient and caregiver satisfaction	Alignment with patient and caregiver choice, preferences, and values
Equity	Equity	Equity	Low variation in access and quality by sociodemographic characteristics
Feasibility	Cost	Efficiency	Cost per unit of improvement
		Financing	Viability and sustainability of funding
	Implementation	Legal feasibility	Feasibility under current laws or regulations or support for new legislation or regulations
		Political feasibility	Support from stakeholder groups
		Operational feasibility	Ease of and capacity for implementation
		Time frame	Speed of implementation

that may not be compatible with others. Appendix D (the appendixes are available at www.rand.org/t/RR597 under the download tab) contains detailed descriptions of the policy options, the rationale for each policy option based on the two key questions we asked the stakeholders, and our evaluation of the policy options on the 14 criteria.

Each policy option has been assigned a number, which does not reflect priority status. Rather, these numbers provide linkages across the report for easy identification.

Table 2.3
Stakeholder-Identified Policy Options for Dementia LTSS Service Delivery

Number	Policy Option	Description
Service Delivery		
SD.1	Minimize transitions and improve coordination of care across providers, settings, and stages of dementia.	Establish standards for coordination of formal and family care, settings, and workforce; use navigators as LTSS counselors (navigators provide counsel on understanding a diagnosis, what treatments are available, and finding and enrolling for services); address access, quality, and outcomes challenges; have all facilities assess cognitive function and allow the assessments to travel with patients across care settings; change reimbursement to encourage providers to work together on transitions; and establish communications channels between care settings and providers.
SD.2	Identify persons with dementia jointly with their family caregivers during emergent, acute, and post-acute care.	Use patient identification bracelets in emergency, acute, and post-acute care settings that identify the patient's family caregiver. Create a field in all electronic medical records and electronic health records to identify a family caregiver.
SD.3	Use patient monitoring technology to assist in dementia LTSS.	Use technology to monitor persons with dementia to prevent wandering or to alter care when health biomarkers (e.g., high blood sugar) indicate a problem.
SD.4	Integrate web- and other technology-based services into dementia LTSS.	Expand telemedicine and online web resources to hard-to-reach populations. Incorporate nurse consultations, medication management (such as electronic pill boxes), imaging consults, and other technology solutions.
SD.5	Create specialized and targeted outreach and education programs for the public, caregivers, professional services organizations, and persons with younger-onset dementia.	Encourage public recognition of signs and symptoms and reduce stigma associated with dementia through the use of specialized outreach and education programs.
SD.6	Standardize complementary assessment tools for persons with dementia and their family caregivers.	Refocus patient assessments on excellence while maintaining minimum safety; standardize patient assessments across stages of dementia, care settings, and states; link patient and caregiver assessments together; and identify quality and health outcomes standards for family caregivers. Involve the National Quality Forum in the standardization of universal quality measures for patients and caregivers. May be paired with SD.7.
SD.7	Encourage the use of quality measurement to ensure consistent use of assessment tools for persons with dementia and their family caregivers.	Adopt quality measures that assess the use of complementary assessment tools for the patient and caregiver pair. Administer complementary assessment tools separately where appropriate. Fund an Institute of Medicine report on family caregiving to address adoption and diffusion challenges for a joint assessment tool. May be paired with SD.6 and SD.11.
SD.8	Establish new and expand existing home- and community-based services.	Establish new and expand existing HCBS that can support persons with dementia in their homes. May be paired with F.8 and F.9.

Table 2.3—continued

Number	Policy Option	Description
SD.9	Expand financial incentives for bundled home, community, and institutional services.	Expand incentives through managed care, accountable care organization networks for LTSS, shared savings from integrating HCBS and LTSS, and bundled care management. Payment models should provide incentives to meet standards of excellence, not just minimum safety expectations. Plan for adaptation and scaling up of bundled payment operations (similar to those used by the Program of All-Inclusive Care for the Elderly [PACE]) to focus on LTSS options.
SD.10	Establish Centers of Excellence models for dementia residential care through the end of life.	Reduce regulatory barriers to innovation and experimentation in assisted living and nursing home care. Create plans to replicate, translate, and scale successful innovations. Revisit the impact of the Olmstead Act (which requires that assisted living and nursing home residents live in minimally restrictive and maximally integrated settings) on persons with dementia. Reassessing these restrictions on dementia care units could facilitate housing persons with dementia together to allow safe wandering in a secure space.
SD.11	Encourage providers' use of cognitive assessment tools for early dementia detection and recognition.	Increase providers' recognition of early signs of cognitive impairment. Encourage utilization of an annual cognitive assessment as part of wellness visits for all Medicare beneficiaries. Establish provider incentives and education to increase use of these tools. May be paired with SD.7.
SD.12	Increase funding for and expand the National Family Caregiver Support Program.	Increase funding under the Older Americans Act for the National Family Caregiver Support Program. Include nonspouse caregivers in the provision of nutrition services.
SD.13	Pass legislation and introduce interventions on Physician Orders for Life-Sustaining Treatments (POLST).	Expand the use of provider orders for life-sustaining treatments. Pass POLST legislation in states where it does not exist and introduce interventions where POLST programs exist to increase penetration in care settings. Make these orders durable across settings and states.
SD.14	Relax the six-month prognosis requirement for hospice care.	Allow patients and their caregivers to request and get hospice care prior to a six-month prognosis. May be paired with F.10.
SD.15	Establish cross-setting teams for persons with dementia, focused on returning the person to the community.	Shorten the duration of nursing home stays by establishing community-, residential-, and institution-based teams focused on returning patients to community and home settings.

NOTE: For more detailed descriptions and additional information on each policy option, see Appendix D (the appendixes are available at www.rand.org/t/RR597 under the download tab).

Table 2.4
Stakeholder-Identified Policy Options for Dementia LTSS Workforce

Number	Policy Option	Description
Workforce		
Formal Caregivers		
W.1	Create new and disseminate existing dementia best practices and training programs for professional and paraprofessional care workers.	Improve dementia-specific training and education of current formal caregivers on communication, care, and referrals. Provide on-the-job training for professional and paraprofessional care workers on how to communicate with, care for, and interact with persons with dementia. Identify opportunities to link families of persons with dementia with appropriate resources.
W.2	Provide specialized geriatric training to direct care professionals while in school.	Require geriatric and behavior management training in medical schools. Require dementia care and geriatrics training in all clinical education. Create specialties within care sectors (e.g., certified nursing assistant for dementia). Expand availability of dementia-specific elective courses in medical and nursing schools.
W.3	Require minimum training and staffing levels at nursing homes and assisted living facilities.	Establish new education, training, and staffing requirements in nursing homes and assisted living facilities. Establish minimum education levels for nursing home and assisted living leaders. Require a registered nurse on site at all times to manage nursing staff, and require minimum training levels for nursing assistants. Require an adequate number of staff per patient. Require consistent staffing patterns. May be paired with W.4.
W.4	Create new and improve existing incentives for the direct care workforce.	Encourage the expansion of the direct care workforce. Decrease staff turnover by improving job satisfaction through higher salaries and more paid time off. Enhance worker safety. Establish loan repayment programs for education in specific subject areas, such as geriatrics. May be paired with W.3.
W.5	Expand nurse delegation laws in all states.	Expand nurse delegation programs across states and increase the number of procedures that may be delegated to caregivers who are not nurses.
Family Caregivers		
W.6	Expand financial compensation programs to family caregivers.	Expand family caregiver compensation programs for lost wages and caregiving work. Increase availability of compensation (e.g., through Medicaid programs) and expand to all states.
W.7	Provide dementia-specific training and information about resources to family caregivers and volunteer groups.	Disseminate educational materials on providing care, hands-on training, and information about respite care, community services, and other resources.
W.8	Expand family-friendly workplace policies.	Expand family-friendly workplace policies nationwide. Offer flexible work hours and paid time off for family caregiving. Expand the Family and Medical Leave Act to cover paid time off and care provided to parents, grandparents, siblings, and others. May be paired with W.9 and W.10.

Table 2.4—continued

Number	Policy Option	Description
W.9	Offer business and individual tax incentives to provide family caregiving.	Include tax breaks for businesses with adult day care centers, flexible spending accounts, paid time off, flexible work hours, and other programs targeting patients and their families with long-term care needs. May be paired with W.8.
W.10	Introduce navigators to provide information on dementia medical care and LTSS.	Introduce employer-sponsored navigators to help employees enroll in and access medical care and long-term care, and receive support. Alternatively, introduce this resource through a government agency. May be paired with W.8.

NOTE: For more detailed descriptions and additional information on each policy option, see Appendix D (the appendixes are available at www.rand.org/t/RR597 under the download tab).

Table 2.5
Stakeholder-Identified Policy Options for Dementia LTSS Financing

Number	Policy Option	Description
Financing		
LTSS Financing		
F.1	Create a national, voluntary opt-out LTC insurance program through a public-private partnership.	Create a national, voluntary opt-out LTC insurance program financed through private insurance premiums. Establish government-sponsored reinsurance for catastrophic loss. Use this program to offer cash benefits. May not be compatible with F.2.
F.2	Adopt a national single-payer LTC insurance system.	Finance a national single-payer LTC insurance program through taxes. The LTSS benefit could be a basic package or comprehensive coverage built into Medicare or a new program. While LTC insurance coverage would be funded through the government, services could be provided by private organizations and other contractors. May not be compatible with F.1.
F.3	Reduce uncertainty in expected returns for private LTC insurance companies.	Encourage private LTC insurance companies to reenter the market. Reduce uncertainty in expected returns for LTC insurance companies by allowing premium increases or by restraining the authority of state insurance commissioners to reject premium increases. Establish a uniform approach to pricing of premiums across all 50 states and territories. May be paired with F.11.
F.4	Link private LTC insurance to reverse mortgage products, other assets, and disability or life insurance products.	Increase public opportunities to consider and get information about LTC insurance options by combining private LTC insurance with other products, such as reverse mortgage products, other assets, or life insurance.
F.5	Link private LTC insurance to health insurance.	Offer private opt-out LTC insurance by combining it with health insurance. Offer this combination both in employer-sponsored health plans and in plans available on health exchanges.

Table 2.5—continued

Number	Policy Option	Description
F.6	Simplify private LTC insurance products.	Simplify LTC insurance products to promote consumer understanding, enable consumer choice, and reduce barriers to LTC insurance uptake. Reduce barriers in the application process and jargon in policies.
F.7	Adopt a capitated payment system for LTSS.	Shift the current fee-for-service LTSS system to capitated payment. Offer risk adjustments and establish quality benchmarks in capitated payment systems.
Medicaid Improvement		
F.8	Broaden Medicaid HCBS waiver programs, self-directed services, and states' infrastructures.	Provide Medicaid benefits for short-term care in assisted living facilities and nursing homes. Encourage the use of programs that pay family members to care for individuals—e.g., cash and counseling or consumer-directed programs. Invest in state Medicaid infrastructures and staff to help people with dementia and their families navigate the system. Invest in state infrastructures and staff training to better support the expansion of Medicaid HCBS waivers. May be paired with SD.8.
F.9	Include HCBS and managed care in state Medicaid plans.	Eliminate the need to apply for waivers by incorporating HCBS and managed care options into state Medicaid plans. May be paired with SD.8.
Medicare Improvement		
F.10	Refine Medicare post-acute care and hospice benefits.	Extend coverage for skilled nursing facility care to include patients who have hospitalization and observation lasting three days. Allow payments for adult day care instead of nursing home care. Extend the definition of *homebound* to include persons with dementia, and include dementia care as a skilled event in home health care. Revise the six-month qualifying requirement for hospice care applicable for persons with dementia. May be paired with SD.14.
Individual Planning and Savings		
F.11	Promote private LTC insurance through education and awareness campaigns.	Increase public awareness and demand for LTC insurance by investing in education and awareness campaigns and by linking LTC and retirement plans. May be paired with F.3.
F.12	Allow individuals to make tax-advantaged contributions for future LTSS expenses.	Encourage individuals to plan early for future LTSS needs and commit future wage increases to savings. Amend Internal Revenue Service Section 529 to help families finance care through HCBS. The Achieving a Better Life Experience Act (ABLE Act), a proposed subsection to Section 529, allows individuals with disabilities, including dementia, to make tax-deferred contributions that can be used for LTSS delivered through HCBS. May be paired with F.13.
F.13	Provide state tax incentives to purchase private LTC insurance.	Expand availability of state tax credits or tax deductions to subsidize individual purchase of private LTC insurance. May be paired with F.12.

NOTE: For more detailed descriptions and additional information on each policy option, see Appendix D (the appendixes are available at www.rand.org/t/RR597 under the download tab).

Comparison of Policy Options to Recommendations in Other Reports

Table 2.6 presents a comparison of the 38 stakeholder-identified policy options to the *National Plan to Address Alzheimer's Disease* and published policy reports from the Alzheimer's Foundation of America and the Commission on Long-Term Care. Of the 38 policy options, 13 (34 percent) overlapped with at least two reports, although no policy options were in agreement across all four reports. The overlapping policy options in the service delivery domain were generally about care coordination, universal assessment tools, expansion of HCBS availability, and establishing care models. Overlapping policy options in the workforce domain were generally about specialized dementia training, meaningful career paths for direct care workers, and training to family caregivers. Overlapping policy options in the financing domain were about expanding Medicaid HCBS waiver programs, broadening eligibility of Medicare post-acute care benefits, and encouraging individual savings.

Ten policy options, identified in Table 2.6 with purple shading, were not included in any of the four comparison plans or reports. This may be due to the fact that the National Plan is focused primarily on activities led by federal agencies, and action steps in the National Plan tend to be national in scope. By contrast, our approach focused on stakeholder-identified policy options and considered national, subnational, and community-based needs at the intersection of dementia and LTSS. Although these ten options are not included in any national report, they may be aligned with policy options described in state-level plans. For example, some state dementia plans[92-94] have recommended tax incentives for individuals who purchase private LTC insurance, which concurs with policy option F.13.

The service delivery options unique to our report reflect dementia's progressive nature, behavioral symptoms that may require more use of technologies that facilitate monitoring and easier access to providers, the strong dependence of persons with dementia on family caregivers, and emphasis on end-of-life care, given its late onset in life.

Workforce dementia LTSS options that were not highlighted in prior national plans focus on increased financial compensation for all family caregivers and helping family caregivers better understand and navigate LTSS.

The National Plan does not contain actions to improve LTSS financing, and the Commission on Long-Term Care was not able to reach consensus on a broad financing solution in the time frame allowed. In addition to dementia LTSS policy options for broad financing solutions that are similar to approaches suggested by the commission, we identified financing options that are complementary but smaller steps in addressing the financing of LTSS. In sum, stakeholders identified unique financing options under a dementia LTSS lens that reflect the concerns about high costs associated with dementia LTSS for federal and state governments and for persons with dementia and their caregivers across all classes of wealth, as well as the need for financial planning and potential linkages with Medicare.

Table 2.6
Map of Policy Options to National Plans and Reports

Number	Dementia LTSS Policy Option	National Plan, 2013[82]	AFA Report, 2012[31]	Commission on Long-Term Care	
				Report, 2013[32]	Alternative Report, 2013[33]
Service Delivery					
SD.1	Minimize transitions and improve coordination of care across providers, settings, and stages of dementia.	■			■
SD.2	Identify persons with dementia jointly with their family caregivers during emergent, acute, and post-acute care.			■	■
SD.3	Use patient monitoring technology to assist in dementia LTSS.				
SD.4	Integrate web- and other technology-based services into dementia LTSS.			■	
SD.5	Create specialized and targeted outreach and education programs for the public, caregivers, professional services organizations, and persons with younger-onset dementia.	■			
SD.6	Standardize complementary assessment tools for persons with dementia and their family caregivers.		■	■	■
SD.7	Encourage the use of quality measurement to ensure consistent use of assessment tools for persons with dementia and their family caregivers.	■	■	■	■
SD.8	Establish new and expand existing HCBS.		■		
SD.9	Expand financial incentives for bundled home, community, and institutional services.		■	■	
SD.10	Establish Centers of Excellence models for dementia residential care through the end of life.		■		
SD.11	Encourage providers' use of cognitive assessment tools for early dementia detection and recognition.	■	■		
SD.12	Increase funding for and expand the National Family Caregiver Support Program.		■		
SD.13	Pass legislation and introduce interventions on POLST.				
SD.14	Relax the six-month prognosis requirement for hospice care.				

Table 2.6—continued

Number	Dementia LTSS Policy Option	National Plan, 2013[82]	AFA Report, 2012[31]	Commission on Long-Term Care	
				Report, 2013[32]	Alternative Report, 2013[33]
SD.15	Establish cross-setting teams for persons with dementia, focused on returning the person to the community.				

Workforce

Formal Caregivers

Number	Dementia LTSS Policy Option	National Plan, 2013[82]	AFA Report, 2012[31]	Report, 2013[32]	Alternative Report, 2013[33]
W.1	Create new and disseminate existing dementia best practices and training programs for professional and paraprofessional care workers.	■			
W.2	Provide specialized geriatric training to direct care professionals while in school.		■		
W.3	Require minimum training and staffing levels at nursing homes and assisted living facilities.	■			
W.4	Create new and improve existing incentives for the direct care workforce.		■	■	■
W.5	Expand nurse delegation laws in all states.			■	

Family Caregivers

W.6	Expand financial compensation to family caregivers.	■			
W.7	Provide dementia-specific training and information about available resources to family caregivers and volunteer groups.	■		■	■
W.8	Expand family-friendly workplace policies.		■		
W.9	Offer business and individual tax incentives to promote family caregiving.		■		
W.10	Introduce navigators to provide information on dementia medical care and LTSS.				

Financing

LTSS Financing

| F.1 | Create a national, voluntary opt-out LTC insurance program through a public-private partnership. | | ■ | | |
| F.2 | Adopt a national single-payer LTC insurance system. | | | * | |

Table 2.6—continued

Number	Dementia LTSS Policy Option	National Plan, 2013[82]	AFA Report, 2012[31]	Commission on Long-Term Care	
				Report, 2013[32]	Alternative Report, 2013[33]
F.3	Reduce uncertainty in expected returns for private LTC insurance companies.			*	
F.4	Link private LTC insurance to reverse mortgage products, other assets, and disability or life insurance products.			*	
F.5	Link private LTC insurance to health insurance.				
F.6	Simplify private LTC insurance products.			▓	
F.7	Adopt a capitated payment system for LTSS.				
Medicaid Improvement					
F.8	Broaden Medicaid HCBS waiver programs, self-directed services, and states' infrastructures.	▓			▓
F.9	Include HCBS and managed care in state Medicaid plans.				
Medicare Improvement					
F.10	Refine Medicare post-acute care and hospice benefits.			▓	▓
Individual Planning and Savings					
F.11	Promote private LTC insurance through education and awareness campaigns.	▓			
F.12	Allow individuals to make tax-advantaged contributions for future LTSS expenses.			▓	▓
F.13	Provide state tax incentives to purchase private LTC insurance.				

* A shaded box with a white asterisk represents an alternative approach in the report, not a recommendation.

NOTE: Family caregivers are defined broadly and include informal caregivers who are relatives, partners, friends, or neighbors who have a significant relationship with, and who provide a broad range of assistance for, an older adult or an adult with chronic or disabling conditions.[17]

Research Directions

The primary objective of this report was to identify and evaluate policy options. As a byproduct of our stakeholder discussions, five priorities for future research were also identified (Table 2.7). These research options should be undertaken to support the implementation of policy options outlined in this blueprint. There are many research gaps that need to be explored at the intersection of dementia and LTSS, and these research directions were identified by stakeholders as the most urgent research priorities that should be addressed immediately in order to remove barriers to implementing policy options. However, these research directions represent only a subset of the potentially long list of many potential research priorities that could be identified in a more systematic look at research gaps. These options should therefore be considered in light of other potential research gaps and the availability of research funds.

Table 2.7
Research Directions

Research Direction	Description
Service Delivery	
Invest in applied research programs on service delivery.	Expand applied research grant programs to improve service delivery. A person-centered outcomes research program is needed to identify the right care for an individual patient at the right time.
Workforce	
Invest in research on the costs, and quality, of dementia care provided through nurse delegation.	Promote research on nurse delegation costs, effects on the gray market (unscreened, unsupervised, and usually untrained workers), and effects on the quality of care provided. Additional research may involve quantifying the costs associated with the absence of new or expanded nurse delegation programs, identifying how many family caregivers cannot work outside the home because they cannot pay a nurse to administer tasks, or understanding how costs borne by family caregivers and the federal or state government may be reduced through nurse delegation.
Financing	
Invest in research on LTSS financing solutions.	Support research on financing solutions. Additional research may be on LTSS costs, the distribution of costs (particularly the amount that is borne by families), how families finance out-of-pocket spending, the impact of changing demographics, and the projected need for LTSS in the future.
Invest in research on the impact of Medicare reforms on dementia care.	Generate evidence on the impact of Medicare changes to eligibility and qualifying events for post-acute care and hospice benefits. This research direction would inform potential changes to Medicare, such as those detailed in policy option F.10.
Invest in research on uptake of private LTC insurance and on consumer understanding of Health Insurance Portability and Accountability Act (HIPAA) tax incentives.	Build evidence on why LTC insurance uptake is low and why HIPAA tax incentives are not optimally used. Research in these areas would help policymakers design better LTC insurance plans and incentive structures to promote the purchase of LTC insurance.

Federal and state policymakers, as well as principal investigators, are the primary stakeholders responsible for pursuing these research directions. Principal investigators are researchers and research funders who set research and evaluation agendas. Further efforts to set priorities for research directions should undertake a stakeholder-engaged process to prioritize research needs, much like those conducted previously for long-term care research topics.[34]

Summary

In this chapter, we presented the methods and results of RAND's stakeholder-engaged policy identification process. We interviewed 30 people representing a variety of stakeholders at the intersection of dementia and LTSS. We asked stakeholders to identify challenges they face in providing care to persons with dementia and their family caregivers and to describe policy options that could be undertaken to address those challenges.

We presented 38 policy options related to service delivery, workforce policy, and financing that were identified by our stakeholders. We also presented a comparison of the policy options with the *National Plan to Address Alzheimer's Disease* and three reports on dementia care or LTSS. Of the 38 policy options, 13 (34 percent) overlapped with at least two reports, although none of the policy options overlapped with all four reports on either dementia or LTSS, reflecting the unique nature of dementia LTSS policy options.

Stakeholders identified ten policy options that did not appear in the four national reports and that are unique to our report. These ten options generally focused on topics that highlight challenges that may be exacerbated for dementia, including its progressive condition; the presence of difficult-to-manage behavioral symptoms; the strong dependence on family caregivers, who require better support; and higher LTSS costs that emphasize the need for financial planning.

We briefly presented our methods for evaluating policy options identified by the stakeholders against 14 evaluation criteria grouped into three domains. These domains were (1) impact—the impact of each policy option on LTSS, (2) equity—the effects of each policy option on equity among subgroups, and (3) feasibility—the feasibility of implementing each policy option. The next and final chapter of the report presents RAND's summary of the evaluations that RAND conducted for each of the 38 policy options, along with our blueprint for the highest-impact policy options that stakeholders may consider to improve dementia LTSS.

CHAPTER THREE

RAND Policy Evaluation and Blueprint Recommendations

Overview

A simultaneous, comprehensive comparison of all 38 policy options on 14 evaluation dimensions and seven stakeholder groups is extremely challenging. Nevertheless, consideration of all of these options, evaluation dimensions, and stakeholder groups is valuable. In this chapter, we synthesize the comprehensive evaluation presented in Chapter Two in order to lay out a blueprint of priority policy options for stakeholders to consider.

The chapter is organized in three sections. First, we evaluate the impact and implementation feasibility for each of the 38 policy options. More detailed summaries of all 38 policy options and our evaluation of them on all 14 impact and feasibility metrics are provided in Appendix D (the appendixes are available at www.rand.org/t/RR597 under the download tab).

Second, we discuss the subset of 25 policy options with the highest impact. These 25 policy options represent RAND's recommendations for the priority policy options that should be pursued to improve dementia LTSS. Our recommendations should be assessed by a larger group of stakeholders and experts—by different stakeholder groups in public proceedings—to identify a shared path toward implementation of improvements in LTSS for persons with dementia.

Third, we provide our recommendations for grouping these high-impact policy options by the stakeholder groups that would have primary responsibility for implementing them. The purpose of this section is to assist stakeholders and experts in organizing a plan of action.

Impact and Feasibility Ratings of Policy Options

To summarize each policy option's impact and feasibility, we subjectively rated a policy option "high impact" if impact stoplight ratings were more frequently green than red (stoplight ratings are included in Appendix D; the appendixes are available at www.rand.org/t/RR597 under the download tab). Similarly, we rated options "high feasibility" if feasibility ratings were more frequently green than red. To assess priorities using this scheme, we did not incorporate information about equity, but we do recommend that in future evaluations, stakeholders consider how a policy affects quality and outcomes for different populations. As one component of impact or feasibility may be more important than other metrics, we subjectively upweighted or downweighted certain metrics if research evidence suggested strong or more direct linkages between the policy option and a metric.

Priority Policy Options for Dementia LTSS

We recommend that the 25 highest-impact policy options (Table 3.1) should be considered for implementation immediately. These high-impact options could be prioritized over feasibility because barriers to implementation can sometimes change relatively quickly as administrations and political environments change, and every effort should be made to reduce or eliminate them. Although our evaluation resulted in 25 priority policy options, many options cannot be pursued in isolation from others and must be bundled to optimize successful implementation and maximum impact on access, quality, and utilization of LTSS. One exception in which options conflict with each other and cannot be undertaken simultaneously is the two national LTSS financing system options. These options outline either creation of a national, voluntary opt-out LTC insurance public-private partnership program or adoption of a national single-payer LTC insurance system. In this case, both options were deemed as having high impact on dementia LTSS, but more research is needed to understand which of the two priority options is most feasible, for example, from a political standpoint. The 25 high-impact policy options are organized into five objectives:

Objective 1: Increase public awareness of dementia to reduce stigma and promote earlier detection.
Objective 2: Improve access to and utilization of LTSS for persons with dementia.
Objective 3: Promote high-quality, person- and family caregiver–centered care.
Objective 4: Provide better support for family caregivers of people with dementia.
Objective 5: Reduce the burden of dementia LTSS costs on individuals and families.

Policy Options by Stakeholders and Stages of Dementia

Meeting each objective requires efforts across multiple sectors and by numerous stakeholders. Thus, Table 3.1 also presents the stakeholder groups primarily responsible for implementing the high-impact policy options.

Table 3.1
25 High-Impact Policy Options for Dementia LTSS

Policy Option	Primary Stakeholders Responsible	Domain
Objective 1: Increase public awareness of dementia to reduce stigma and promote earlier detection of signs and symptoms.		
Create specialized and targeted outreach and education programs for the public, caregivers, professional services organizations, and persons with younger-onset dementia.	Providers—formal Policymakers—fed, st, loc	SD
Encourage providers' use of cognitive assessment tools for early dementia detection and recognition.	Providers—formal Policymakers—fed, st, loc Principal investigators	SD
Objective 2: Improve access to and utilization of LTSS for persons with dementia.		
Establish new and expand existing HCBS.	Providers—formal Policymakers—fed, st	SD
Integrate web- and other technology-based services into dementia LTSS.	Providers—formal Policymakers—fed, st Product makers	SD
Create new and improve existing incentives for the direct care workforce.	Providers—formal Policymakers—fed, st, loc	W
Expand nurse delegation laws in all states.	Policymakers—fed, st	W
Broaden Medicaid HCBS waiver programs, self-directed services, and states' infrastructures.	Payers—public Policymakers—fed, st	F
Include HCBS and managed care in state Medicaid plans.	Payers—public Policymakers—st	F
Refine Medicare post-acute care and hospice benefits.	Payers—public Policymakers—fed	F
Objective 3: Promote high-quality, person- and family caregiver–centered care.		
Establish Centers of Excellence models for dementia residential care through the end of life.	Providers—formal Payers—public, private Policymakers—fed	SD
Minimize transitions and improve coordination of care across providers, settings, and stages of dementia.	Providers—formal Policymakers—fed, st	SD
Expand financial incentives for bundled home, community, and institutional services.	Providers—formal Payers—public, private Policymakers—fed, st	SD
Establish cross-setting teams for persons with dementia, focused on returning the person to the community.	Providers—formal, family Payers—public, private Policymakers—fed, st	SD
Encourage the use of quality measurement to ensure consistent use of assessment tools for persons with dementia and their family caregivers.	Providers—formal Payers—public, private Policymakers—fed, st	SD

Table 3.1—continued

Policy Option	Primary Stakeholders Responsible	Domain
Identify persons with dementia jointly with their family caregivers during emergent, acute, and post-acute care.	Providers—formal Product makers	SD
Standardize complementary assessment tools for persons with dementia and their family caregivers.	Providers—formal Policymakers—fed, st Principal investigators	SD
Create new and disseminate existing dementia best practices and training programs for professional and paraprofessional care workers.	Providers—formal Policymakers—fed, st, loc	W
Provide specialized geriatric training to direct care professionals while in school.	Providers—formal Policymakers—fed, st, loc	W
Objective 4: Provide better support for family caregivers of people with dementia.		
Provide dementia-specific training and information about resources to family caregivers and volunteer groups.	Providers—formal	W
Offer business and individual tax incentives to promote family caregiving.	Policymakers—fed, st, loc	W
Expand financial compensation programs to family caregivers.	Payers—public, private Policymakers—fed, st	W
Expand family-friendly workplace policies.	Purchasers Policymakers—fed, st, loc	W
Objective 5: Reduce the burden of dementia LTSS costs on individuals and families.		
Link private LTC insurance to health insurance.	Payers—public, private	F
Create a national, voluntary opt-out LTC insurance program through a public-private partnership.	Payers—public, private Policymakers—fed, st	F
Adopt a national single-payer LTC insurance system.	Payers—public Policymakers—fed	F

NOTES: fed = federal, st = state, loc = local, SD = service delivery, W = workforce, and F = financing. Family caregivers are defined broadly and include informal caregivers who are relatives, partners, friends, or neighbors who have a significant relationship with, and who provide a broad range of assistance for, an older adult or an adult with chronic or disabling conditions.[17] Principal investigators include researchers and research funders.

Tables D.7–D.9 in Appendix D (the appendixes are available at www.rand.org/t/ RR597 under the download tab) indicate the primary and secondary stakeholders responsible, as well as the stakeholders affected, for all policy options. This assignment may help stakeholders consider resource allocation and prioritization, as well as partnerships to work hand in hand to implement policy options. The stakeholders are grouped according to the 7Ps framework: patients and public, providers, purchasers, payers, policymakers, product makers, and principal investigators (Table 2.1). Stakeholders responsible for carrying out the 25 priority policy options were primarily providers, payers, and policymakers. Nonetheless, we indicate the importance of engaging stakeholders who play a supportive role or who would be affected by implementation. Patients and providers are among the stakeholders most likely to be affected by new policy, and they should therefore be engaged even when not designated to implement the policy.

On average, a person with Alzheimer's disease will spend more years in the most severe stage of the disease than in any other stage.[95] Therefore, it is critical to consider strategies by stage of dementia. We use the seven stages of dementia depicted in Appendix Figure D.1 to present how the high-impact policy options align with the stages of dementia in Appendix Table D.10 (the appendixes are available at www.rand.org/t/RR597 under the download tab). Generally, the high-impact policy options are relevant across the dementia continuum. Policy options that are most relevant to the early stages of dementia are related to early diagnosis, providing dementia-specific training providers, increasing access to HCBS, and assisting caregivers and persons with dementia with financial planning. Throughout all stages of dementia, the high-impact policy options focus on quality of care, minimizing transitions in care settings, creating bundled services, and broadening Medicare benefits.

Summary

This blueprint, to our knowledge, is the first to outline stakeholder-based national priority policy options for dementia LTSS. We recommend consideration of 25 high-impact policy options that could be considered for immediate implementation. While these 25 priority policy options may address multiple objectives, they can be broadly summarized into five objectives that fill key gaps in the dementia LTSS system: (1) increase public awareness of dementia to reduce stigma and promote earlier detection; (2) improve access to and utilization of LTSS for persons with dementia; (3) promote high-quality, person- and family caregiver–centered care; (4) provide better support for family caregivers of people with dementia; and (5) reduce the burden of dementia LTSS costs on individuals and families.

These broad objectives address challenges with (1) stigma and early detection of signs and symptoms of dementia that can affect downstream access to and quality of care; (2) inadequate access to and measurement of quality LTSS; (3) fragmented delivery systems that may affect persons with dementia more severely because of the heavy reliance on family caregivers and nonmedical LTSS providers; (4) an undertrained, understaffed, and often inadequately compensated caregiving workforce; and (5) insufficient public and private options to help individuals and their families deal with the costs associated with dementia LTSS. Although our evaluation resulted in recommendations of these 25 policy options, many options cannot be pursued in isolation from others and must be bundled to optimize implementation and impact on access, quality, and utilization of LTSS. One exception in which options conflict with each other and cannot be undertaken simultaneously is the two national LTSS financing system options. In this case, both options were deemed as having high impact on dementia LTSS, but more research is needed to understand which of the two priority options is most feasible, for example, from a political standpoint.

Comparison with Other Dementia or LTSS National Plans and Reports

Our stakeholder-engaged process for creating this blueprint resulted in 38 policy options, 25 of which were rated high-impact. Of the 25, ten options do not appear in other national strategies or plans that are focused individually on LTSS or dementia, but not jointly on LTSS for persons with dementia. Four of the ten unique options identified in this report were also rated among our 25 highest-impact options:

- Establish a joint team for persons with dementia, focused on returning the person to the community.
- Expand financial compensation to family caregivers.
- Link private LTC insurance to health insurance.
- Include home- and community-based services and managed care in state Medicaid plans.

These options are critical to consider in the near term as LTSS system gaps increasingly influence the growing population of persons with dementia.

Strengths and Limitations

The strengths of our study include the engagement of interviewees representing stakeholder perspectives across the health care system, the comparison of policy options with options recommended by other national efforts, and the evaluation and prioritization of policy options. More importantly, this is the only evaluation that places a spotlight on stakeholder-generated policy options in LTSS for dementia specifically. Despite these strengths, we note several limitations.

First, as with many qualitative research studies that interview a selected group of key informants, our research may lack representativeness within the stakeholder groups. The 38 policy options identified through our stakeholder-engagement process are not an exhaustive list, and the policy options may differ from those identified through different strategies, such as systematic reviews, or through wider sampling strategies that might have improved the representativeness of stakeholder groups.

Second, we applied qualitative stoplight ratings to evaluate the 38 options on their impact, feasibility, and equity, but these evaluations were not informed by empirical evidence in every case.

Third, we assessed feasibility of each policy option at one point in time. Feasibility metrics, such as political feasibility, can change in this rapidly evolving field, and policy options that seem infeasible during one period may change with new administrations or cultural shifts.

Finally, all causes of dementia were generally treated as a homogeneous group in this report. However, the policy options may not apply uniformly to dementias with different etiologies (such as younger-onset dementia), which may affect individuals who are still employed, who may be cared for by younger family caregivers, or who have a longer stage for LTSS planning.

Future Steps

These limitations should be addressed in future work in which a larger group of stakeholders is convened to assign strength of evidence metrics to the qualitative impact, feasibility, and equity ratings and reaches a consensus on how best to select and carry out priority policy options. This larger sample of stakeholders may also consider whether policy options may have varied results depending on the types of dementia. Finally, gaps in the qualitative rating approach we used can be filled by conducting systematic literature reviews of evidence-based programs, cost-effectiveness analyses of each policy option, and analyses using existing administrative and clinical data. These types of studies would facilitate a better understanding of the strength of evidence for each rating.

In the process of consensus-building, we recommend that dementia LTSS stakeholders work together to develop metrics or key performance indicators of LTSS system performance for persons affected by dementia in order to monitor progressive improvements on each of the five overarching objectives. Examples of metrics may include

- a target percentage of the estimated population with dementia that has received a diagnosis
- a target percentage of the Medicaid-eligible diagnosed population that has a quality care plan and is receiving desired HCBS
- cross-setting teams and person-centered care plans for a target percentage of persons with diagnosed dementia
- dementia-specific training received by a target proportion of family caregivers within a specific time frame following a diagnosis

- a target percentage reduction in median out-of-pocket dementia LTSS costs for persons with dementia and their families.

Process metrics may also be measured, including the extent of communication between stakeholders, the number of panel roundtable discussions that take place, the amount of research funding allocated to determine data sources, the establishment of monitoring plans for meeting metrics, and the adoption of responsibility for taking action on metrics by stakeholders across multiple sectors.

In conclusion, it is our hope that this research will highlight the need for stakeholders to focus on dementia LTSS policies and will serve as the foundation for a larger group of stakeholders to build consensus around the dementia LTSS policy options that should be pursued most urgently.

References[1]

[1] Hurd MD, Martorell P, Delavande A, Mullen KJ, and Langa KM, "Monetary Costs of Dementia in the United States," *New England Journal of Medicine*, Vol. 368, No. 14, 2013, pp. 1326–1334.

[2] Alzheimer's Association, *2013 Alzheimer's Disease Facts and Figures*, 2013.

[3] Hoyert DL and Xu J, *Deaths: Preliminary Data for 2011*, Hyattsville, Md.: National Center for Health Statistics, 2012.

[4] National Institutes of Health, *The Dementias: Hope Through Research*, 2013.

[5] Alzheimer's Association, "2014 Alzheimer's Disease Facts and Figures," *Alzheimer's & Dementia*, Vol. 10, No. 2, 2014.

[6] Murray CJ, Abraham J, Ali MK, et al. (US Burden of Disease Collaborators), "The State of US Health, 1990–2010: Burden of Diseases, Injuries, and Risk Factors," *Journal of the American Medical Association*, Vol. 310, No. 6, 2013, pp. 591–606.

[7] Harris-Kojetin L, Sengupta M, Park-Lee E, and Valverde R, *Long-Term Care Services in the United States: 2013 Overview*, Hyattsville, Md.: National Center for Health Statistics, 2013.

[8] World Health Organization, *Dementia: A Public Health Priority*, United Kingdom, 2012.

[9] Boustani M, Peterson B, Hanson L, Harris R, and Lohr KN, "Screening for Dementia in Primary Care: A Summary of the Evidence for the U.S. Preventive Services Task Force," 2003. As of May 9, 2014:
http://www.uspreventiveservicestaskforce.org/3rduspstf/dementia/dementsum.htm

[10] U.K. Department of Health, *Dementia: A State of the Nation Report on Dementia Care and Support in England*, 2013.

[11] Carpenter B and Dave J, "Disclosing a Dementia Diagnosis: A Review of Opinion and Practice, and a Proposed Research Agenda," *The Gerontologist*, Vol. 44, No. 2, 2004, pp. 149–158.

[12] Robinson L, Clare L, and Evans K, "Making Sense of Dementia and Adjusting to Loss: Psychological Reactions to a Diagnosis of Dementia in Couples," *Aging & Mental Health*, Vol. 9, No. 4, 2005, pp. 337–347.

[13] Georges J and Gove D, "Disclosing a Diagnosis: The Alzheimer Europe View," *Journal of Dementia Care*, Vol. 15, No. 6, 2007, pp. 28–29.

---

[1] These references are also available in alphabetical order in the appendixes to this report. The appendixes are available at www.rand.org/t/RR597 under the download tab.

[14] Laakkonen M, Raivio M, Eloniemi-Sulkava U, Saarenheimo M, Pietilä M, Tilvis RS, and Pitkälä KH, "How Do Elderly Spouse Care Givers of People with Alzheimer Disease Experience the Disclosure of Dementia Diagnosis and Subsequent Care?" *Journal of Medical Ethics*, Vol. 34, No. 6, 2008, pp. 427–430.

[15] Ng T, Harrington C, Musumeci M, and Reaves EL, *Medicaid Home and Community-Based Services Programs: 2010 Data Update*, Washington, D.C.: Kaiser Family Foundation, 2014.

[16] Redfoot D, Feinberg L, and Houser A, *The Aging of the Baby Boom and the Growing Care Gap: A Look at Future Declines in the Availability of Family Caregivers*, Washington, D.C., 2013.

[17] Feinberg L, Reinhard SC, Houser A, and Choula R, *Valuing the Invaluable: 2011 Update: The Growing Contributions and Costs of Family Caregiving*, Washington, D.C., 2011.

[18] AARP, The Commonwealth Fund, and the SCAN Foundation, "Raising Expectations: A State Scorecard on Long-Term Services and Supports for Older Adults, People with Physical Disabilities, and Family Caregivers," 2014. As of February 26, 2014:
http://www.longtermscorecard.org/

[19] National Alliance for Caregiving and AARP, *Caregiving in the U.S. Executive Summary*, 2009.

[20] Gibson AK and Anderson KA, "Difficult Diagnoses: Family Caregivers' Experiences During and Following the Diagnostic Process for Dementia," *American Journal of Alzheimer's Disease and Other Dementias*, Vol. 26, No. 3, 2011, pp. 212–217.

[21] Laakkonen ML, Raivio MM, Eloniemi-Sulkava U, Tilvis RS, and Pitkälä KH, "Disclosure of Dementia Diagnosis and the Need for Advance Care Planning in Individuals with Alzheimer's Disease," *Journal of the American Geriatrics Society*, Vol. 56, No. 11, 2008, pp. 2156–2157.

[22] National Association of State Units on Aging, *Nursing Home Abuse Risk Prevention Profile and Checklist*, Washington, D.C.: National Center on Elder Abuse, 2005.

[23] Spilsbury K, Hewitt C, Stirk L, and Bowman C, "The Relationship Between Nurse Staffing and Quality of Care in Nursing Homes: A Systematic Review," *International Journal of Nursing Studies*, Vol. 48, No. 6, 2011, pp. 732–750.

[24] Reuben DB, Bachrach PS, McCreath H, Simpson D, Bragg EJ, Warshaw GA, Snyder R, and Frank JC, "Changing the Course of Geriatrics Education: An Evaluation of the First Cohort of Reynolds Geriatrics Education Programs," *Academic Medicine: Journal of the Association of American Medical Colleges*, Vol. 84, No. 5, 2009, p. 619.

[25] Warshaw GA and Bragg EJ, "Preparing the Health Care Workforce to Care for Adults with Alzheimer's Disease and Related Dementias," *Health Affairs*, Vol. 33, No. 4, 2014, pp. 633–641.

[26] Federal Interagency Forum on Aging-Related Statistics, *Older Americans 2012: Key Indicators of Well-Being*, Washington, D.C.: U.S. Government Printing Office, 2012.

[27] SCAN Foundation, *Who Pays for Long-Term Care in the U.S.? (Updated)*, Long Beach, Calif.: SCAN Foundation, 2013.

[28] Alper J, *The Partnership for Long-Term Care: A Public-Private Partnership to Finance Long-Term Care*, Robert Wood Johnson Foundation, 2006.

[29] U.S. Department of Health and Human Services, *National Alzheimer's Project Act*, 2014. As of May 8, 2014:
http://aspe.hhs.gov/daltcp/napa/

[30] U.S. Department of Health and Human Services, *National Plan to Address Alzheimer's Disease: 2013 Update*, 2013. As of May 8, 2014:
http://aspe.hhs.gov/daltcp/napa/NatlPlan2013.pdf

[31] Hall EJ and Sokol EW, *Time to Build: Action Steps and Recommendations to Update the "National Plan to Address Alzheimer's Disease,"* New York, N.Y.: Alzheimer's Foundation of America, 2012.

[32] Commission on Long-Term Care, *Report to the Congress*, Washington, D.C., 2013.

[33] Commission on Long-Term Care, *A Comprehensive Approach to Long-Term Services and Supports*, 2013.

[34] Wysocki A, Butler M, Kane RL, and Shippee T, *Future Research Needs: Long-Term Care for Older Adults*, Rockville, Md.: Agency for Healthcare Research and Quality, 2013.

[35] Burns A and Iliffe S, "Dementia," *BMJ*, Vol. 338, 2009, pp. 405–409.

[36] James BD, Leurgans SE, Hebert LE, Scherr PA, Yaffe K, and Bennett DA, "Contribution of Alzheimer Disease to Mortality in the United States," *Neurology*, Vol. 82, No. 2, 2014, pp. 1045–1050.

[37] Administration on Aging, *A Profile of Older Americans: 2005*, Washington, D.C.: U.S. Department of Health and Human Services, 2007.

[38] Kaye H, Harrington C, and LaPlante M, "Long-Term Care: Who Gets It, Who Provides It, Who Pays, and How Much?" *Health Affairs*, Vol. 29, No. 1, 2010, pp. 11–21.

[39] Alzheimer's Disease International, *Policy Brief for Heads of Government: The Global Impact of Dementia 2013–2050*, London, 2013.

[40] Alzheimer's Association, *Alzheimer's Disease and Chronic Health Conditions: The Real Challenge for 21st Century Medicare*, undated.

[41] Callahan CM, Arling G, Tu W, Rosenman MB, Counsell SR, Stump TE, and Hendrie HC, "Transitions in Care for Older Adults With and Without Dementia," *Journal of the American Geriatrics Society*, Vol. 60, No. 5, 2012, pp. 813–820.

[42] Finn JC, Flicker L, Mackenzie E, Jacobs IG, Fatovich DM, Drummond S, Harris M, Holman DC, and Sprivulis P, "Interface Between Residential Aged Care Facilities and a Teaching Hospital Emergency Department in Western Australia," *Medical Journal of Australia*, Vol. 184, No. 9, 2006, p. 432.

[43] Inouye SK, "The Dilemma of Delirium: Clinical and Research Controversies Regarding Diagnosis and Evaluation of Delirium in Hospitalized Elderly Medical Patients," *American Journal of Medicine*, Vol. 97, 1994, pp. 278–288.

[44] Hagglund M and Scandurra I, "Studying Intersection Points—An Analysis of Information Needs for Shared Homecare of Elderly Patients," *Journal on Information Technology in Healthcare*, Vol. 7, 2007, pp. 23–42.

[45] Gaugler JE, Kane RL, and Kane RA, "Family Care for Older Adults with Disabilities: Toward More Targeted and Interpretable Research," *International Journal of Aging and Human Development*, Vol. 54, No. 3, 2012, pp. 205–231

[46] Lyketsos CG, Toone L, Tschanz J, Rabins PV, Steinberg M, Onyike CU, Corcoran C, Norton M, Zandi P, Breitner JCS, and Welsh-Bohmer K, "Population-Based Study of Medical Comorbidity in Early Dementia and 'Cognitive Impairment, No Dementia (CIND)': Association with Functional and Cognitive Impairment: The Cache County Study," *American Journal of Geriatric Psychiatry*, Vol. 13, No. 8, 2005, pp. 656–664.

[47] Thies W and Bleiler L, "2013 Alzheimer's Disease Facts and Figures," *Alzheimer's & Dementia*, Vol. 9, No. 2, 2013, pp. 208–245.

[48] National Alliance for Caregiving and AARP, *Caregiving in the U.S. Data Analyzed Under Contract for the Alzheimer's Association* (unpublished), 2009.

[49] VandeWeerd C, Paveza GJ, Walsh M, and Corvin J, "Physical Mistreatment in Persons with Alzheimer's Disease," *Journal of Aging Research*, 2013.

[50] Dong X, Chen R, and Simon MA, "Elder Abuse and Dementia: A Review of the Research and Health Policy," *Health Affairs*, Vol. 33, No. 4, 2014, pp. 642–649.

[51] Cooper C, Selwood A, Blanchard M, Walker Z, Blizard R, and Livingston G, "Abuse of People with Dementia by Family Carers: Representative Cross Sectional Survey," *BMJ*, Vol. 338, 2009.

[52] Center of Excellence on Elder Abuse and Neglect, *How at Risk for Abuse Are People with Dementia?* Irvine, Calif.: National Center on Elder Abuse, undated.

[53] Schubert CC, Boustani M, Callahan CM, Perkins AJ, Carney CP, Fox C, Unverzagt F, Hui S, and Hendrie HC, "Comorbidity Profile of Dementia Patients in Primary Care: Are They Sicker?" *Journal of the American Geriatric Society*, Vol. 54, No. 1, 2006, pp. 104–109.

[54] Hill JW, Futterman R, Duttagupta S, Mastey V, Lloyd JR, and Fillit H, "Alzheimer's Disease and Related Dementias Increase Costs of Comorbidities in Managed Medicare," *Neurology*, Vol. 58, No. 1, 2002, pp. 62–70.

[55] Feng Z, Coots LA, Kaganova Y, and Wiener JM, "Hospital and ED Use Among Medicare Beneficiaries with Dementia Varies by Setting and Proximity to Death," *Health Affairs*, Vol. 33, No. 4, 2014, pp. 683–690.

[56] Sloan F and Taylor DJ, "Effect of Alzheimer Disease on the Cost of Treating Other Diseases," *Alzheimer Disease and Associated Disorders*, Vol. 16, 2002, pp. 137–143.

[57] Alzheimer's Association, *2010 Alzheimer's Disease Facts and Figures*, 2010.

[58] Dilworth-Anderson P, Hendrie H, Manly J, Khachaturian A, and Fazio S, "Diagnosis and Assessment of Alzheimer's Disease in Diverse Populations," *Alzheimer's & Dementia*, Vol. 4, 2008, pp. 305–309.

[59] Manly J and Mayeux R, "Ethnic Differences in Dementia and Alzheimer's Disease," in Anderson NB, Bulatao R, and Cohen B, eds., *Critical Perspectives on Racial and Ethnic Differences in Health in Late Life*, Washington, D.C.: National Academies Press, 2004, pp. 95–141.

[60] Alzheimer's Association, "Down Syndrome and Alzheimer's Disease," 2014. As of March 14, 2014: http://www.alz.org/dementia/down-syndrome-alzheimers-symptoms.asp

[61] Robinson L, Gemski A, Abley C, Bond J, Keady J, Campbell S, Samsi K, and Manthorpe J, "The Transition to Dementia—Individual and Family Experiences of Receiving a Diagnosis: A Review," *International Psychogeriatrics*, Vol. 23, No. 7, 2011, pp. 1026–1043.

[62] Alexander GL, Madsen R, and Wakefield D, "A Regional Assessment of Information Technology Sophistication in Missouri Nursing Homes," *Policy, Politics, & Nursing Practice*, Vol. 11, No. 3, 2010, pp. 214–225.

[63] Georgiou A, Marks A, Braithwaite J, and Westbrook JI, "Gaps, Disconnections, and Discontinuities— The Role of Information Exchange in the Delivery of Quality Long-Term Care," *The Gerontologist*, Vol. 53, No. 5, 2013, pp. 770–779.

[64] Banerjee S, Willis R, Matthews D, Contell F, Chan J, and Murray J, "Improving the Quality of Care for Mild to Moderate Dementia: An Evaluation of the Croydon Memory Service Model," *International Journal of Geriatric Psychiatry*, Vol. 22, No. 8, 2007, pp. 782–788.

[65] Bouldin ED and Andresen E, *Caregiving Across the United States: Caregivers of Persons with Alzheimer's Disease or Dementia in 8 States and the District of Columbia, Data from the 2009 & 2010 Behavioral Risk Factor Surveillance System*, 2014.

[66] Family Caregiver Alliance National Center on Caregiving, "Fact Sheet: Caregiver's Guide to Understanding Dementia Behaviors," 2014. As of February 26, 2014:
http://www.caregiver.org/jsp/content_node.jsp?nodeid=391

[67] Ory MG, Hoffman RR III, Yee JL, Tennstedt S, and Schulz R, "Prevalence and Impact of Caregiving: A Detailed Comparison Between Dementia and Nondementia Caregivers," *The Gerontologist*, Vol. 39, No. 2, 1999, pp. 177–185.

[68] Mohide EA, Torrance GW, Streiner DL, Pringle DM, and Gilbert R, "Measuring the Wellbeing of Family Caregivers Using the Time Trade-Off Technique," *Journal of Clinical Epidemiology*, Vol. 41, No. 5, 1988, pp. 475–482.

[69] Cuijpers P, "Depressive Disorders in Caregivers of Dementia Patients: A Systematic Review," *Aging & Mental Health*, Vol. 9, No. 4, 2005, pp. 325–330.

[70] Fisher GG, Franks MM, Plassman BL, Brown SL, Potter GG, Llewellyn D, Rogers MA, and Langa KM, "Caring for Individuals with Dementia and Cognitive Impairment, Not Dementia: Findings from the Aging, Demographics, and Memory Study," *Journal of the American Geriatrics Society*, Vol. 59, No. 3, 2011, pp. 488–494.

[71] Schubert CC, Boustani M, Callahan CM, Perkins AJ, and Hendrie HC, "Acute Care Utilization by Dementia Caregivers Within Urban Primary Care Practices," *Journal of General Internal Medicine*, Vol. 23, No. 11, 2008, pp. 1736–1740.

[72] Schulz R and Beach SR, "Caregiving as a Risk Factor for Mortality: The Caregiver Health Effects Study," *Journal of the American Medical Association*, Vol. 262, 1999, pp. 2215–2219.

[73] Christakis NA and Allison PD, "Mortality After the Hospitalization of a Spouse," *New England Journal of Medicine*, Vol. 354, No. 7, 2006, pp. 719–730.

[74] Llanque SM and Enriquez M, "Interventions for Hispanic Caregivers of Patients with Dementia: A Review of the Literature," *American Journal of Alzheimer's Disease and Other Dementias*, Vol. 27, No. 1, 2012, pp. D3–D32.

[75] Paraprofessional Healthcare Institute, *November 2013 Update*, Bronx, N.Y., 2013.

[76] Menne HL, Ejaz FK, Noelker LS, and Jones JA, "Direct Care Workers' Recommendations for Training and Continuing Education," *Gerontology & Geriatrics Education*, Vol. 28, No. 2, 2007, pp. 91–108.

[77] Stone R, "Testimony Before the Senate Special Committee on Aging," Hearing on Impending Shortages of Health Professionals Trained to Care for Older Adults, 2008.

[78] Institute for the Future of Aging Services, *The Long-Term Care Workforce: Can the Crisis Be Fixed? Problems, Causes and Options*, Washington, D.C.: Institute for the Future of Aging Services, 2007.

[79] Eiken S, Sredl K, Gold L, Kasten J, Burwell B, and Saucier P, *Medicaid Expenditures for Long Term Services and Supports in 2011*, 2013.

[80] Bynum J, *Characteristics, Costs and Health Service Use for Medicare Beneficiaries with a Dementia Diagnosis: Report 1 Medicare Current Beneficiary Survey*, 2009.

[81] U.S. Department of Health and Human Services, *National Plan to Address Alzheimer's Disease*, 2012.

[82] U.S. Department of Health and Human Services, *National Plan to Address Alzheimer's Disease: 2013 Update*, 2013. As of May 8, 2014:
http://aspe.hhs.gov/daltcp/napa/NatlPlan2013.pdf

[83] Sebelius K, Secretary Sebelius' letter to Congress about CLASS, U.S. Department of Health and Human Services, Washington, D.C., 2011.

[84] U.S. Department of Health and Human Services, *A Report on the Actuarial, Marketing, and Legal Analyses of the CLASS Program*, 2011.

[85] California Health Advocates, "CLASS Act Repealed & Federal Long-Term Care Commission Appointed: What's Next?" May 15, 2013. As of February 26, 2014:
http://www.cahealthadvocates.org/news/long-term/2013/
class-act-repealed-federal-long-term-sales-comission%20appointed.html

[86] Alzheimer's Association, "State Plans," 2014. As of February 26, 2014:
http://act.alz.org/site/PageNavigator/state_plans.html

[87] Alzheimer's Association, *State Alzheimer's Disease Plans: State Government Structure*, undated.

[88] Reinhard SC, Kassner E, Houser A, and Mollica R, *Raising Expectations: A State Scorecard on Long-Term Services and Supports for Older Adults, People with Physical Disabilities, and Family Caregivers*, 2011.

[89] Centers for Disease Control and Prevention, "Healthy Brain Initiative," last updated April 1, 2014. As of April 22, 2014:
http://www.cdc.gov/aging/healthybrain/

[90] Concannon TW, Meissner P, Grunbaum JA, McElwee N, Guise JM, Santa J, Conway PH, Daudelin D, Morrato EH, and Leslie LK, "A New Taxonomy for Stakeholder Engagement in Patient-Centered Outcomes Research," *Journal of General Internal Medicine*, Vol. 27, No. 8, 2012, pp. 985–991.

[91] Braun V and Clarke V, "Using Thematic Analysis in Psychology," *Qualitative Research in Psychology*, Vol. 3, No. 2, 2006, pp. 77–101.

[92] Office on Alzheimer's Disease and Related Disorders and Kentucky Alzheimer's Disease and Related Disorders Advisory Council, *Setting a Roadmap to Address Alzheimer's in the Commonwealth: A Report on the Assessment of the Current and Anticipated Future Impact of Alzheimer's Disease and Related Dementias on Kentuckians with Recommendations for Action*, Frankfort, Ky.: Department for Aging and Independent Living, 2008.

[93] Alzheimer's Disease Task Force Members, *Tennessee Alzheimer's Disease Task Force Final Report*, Nashville, Tenn.: Tennessee Commission on Aging and Disability, 2009.

[94] Purple Ribbon Task Force, *Conquering the Specter of Alzheimer's Disease in South Carolina*, Columbia, S.C.: Lt. Governor's Office on Aging, 2009.

[95] Arrighi HM, Neumann PJ, Lieberburg IM, and Townsend RJ, "Lethality of Alzheimer Disease and Its Impact on Nursing Home Placement," *Alzheimer Disease & Associated Disorders*, Vol. 24, No. 1, 2010, pp. 90–95.